THE PATIENT AND DECENTRALIZED TESTING

THE PATIENT AND DECENTRALIZED TESTING

Edited by J. P. Ashby
Department of Clinical Chemistry
Northwick Park Hospital and Clinical Research Centre
Harrow, Middlesex, UK

Proceedings of the ECCLS Conference on Decentralized Clinical Training held in Copenhagen, 11-12th August 1986.

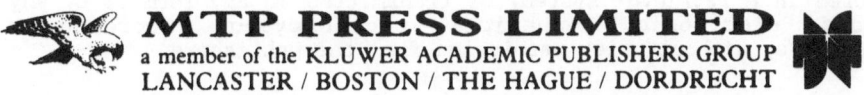

MTP PRESS LIMITED
a member of the KLUWER ACADEMIC PUBLISHERS GROUP
LANCASTER / BOSTON / THE HAGUE / DORDRECHT

Published in the UK and Europe by
MTP Press Limited
Falcon House
Lancaster, England

British Library Cataloguing in Publication Data

The Patient and decentralized testing.
  1. Pathological services.
  I. Ashby, J.P.
  616'.075   RB37

ISBN-13:978-94-010-7926-6   e-ISBN-13:978-94-009-3179-4
DOI: 10.1007/978-94-009-3179-4

Published in the USA by
MTP Press
A division of Kluwer Academic Publishers
101 Philip Drive
Norwell, MA 02061, USA

Library of Congress Cataloging-in-Publication Data

ECCLS Seminar (7th : 1986 : Copenhagen, Denmark)
  The patient and decentralized testing.

  Includes bibliographies and index.
  1. Diagnosis, Laboratory--Congresses. 2. Medical
innovations--Congresses. I. Ashby, J. P. II. Title.
[DNLM: 1. Delivery of Health Care--organizations &
administration--congresses. 2. Diagnosis, Laboratory--
congresses. 3. Technology, Medical--trends--congresses.]
W3 EC12 7th 1986p   616.07'5   87-2737

Contents

Preface FL Mitchell vii

List of Contributors viii

Foreword R Dybkaer x

Welcoming Address JE Asvall xiii

PART 1, WHAT IS THE NEED FOR DECENTRALIZED TESTING?

1 The need for decentralized testing - a patient's view
E Seidenfaden 3
Discussion 8

2 The need for decentralized testing - a general
practitioner's view
P Backer 9

3 The need for decentralized testing - a hospital
clinician's view
P Riis 13

4 The need for decentralized testing - a laboratorian's
view
N Tryding 15
Discussion 20

**PART 2 WHAT IS BEING PROVIDED BY INDUSTRY FOR
DECENTRALIZED TESTING?**

5 Equipment for the side ward, the doctor's premises and the
patient's home
C Kirkemo 23

PART 3 IS THE CHANGED RESPONSIBILITY WELCOME?

6 Is the changed responsibility welcome? A nurse's view
M Locker de Bruijne 33

7 Is the changed responsibility welcome? A laboratorian's
view
G Smart 37
Discussion 40

**PART 4   THE ROLE OF ECCLS IN STANDARDS FOR GOOD PRAC-
TICE IN DECENTRALIZED CLINICAL LABORATORIES**

8   Premises and operational units
     DM Browning   43
     Discussion   47

9   Methods and reagents
     H Küffer   49
     Discussion   53

10   Safety of personnel and environment
     RD Jennings   57
     Discussion   60

11   Patient reception, preparation, specimen handling and
     data flow
     CE Wilde   63
     Discussion   72

12   Quality assurance, teaching and training
     D Kutter   73
     Discussion   83

13   Special considerations in haematology and blood banking
     DW Dawson   85
     Discussion   88

14   Special considerations in histopathology
     N. Stormby   89
     Discussion   91

15   Organization and management in the decentralized
     laboratory
     RM Rowan   93
     Discussion   100

PART 5   COST IMPLICATIONS OF DECENTRALIZED TESTING

16   Cost implications of decentralized testing - a health
     agency's view
     R Netter   105
     Discussion   107

17   Cost implications of decentralized testing - a
     laboratorian's view
     R Haeckel   109
     Discussion   117

PART 6   SUMMARY AND CONCLUSIONS

18   The need for guidelines for decentralized clinical
     testing
     R Dybkaer   121

Preface

For this the seventh and subsequent seminars, the Board of
ECCLS has decided that to maximize local input and generally im-
porve the efficiency of organization, a selected country might be
asked to host a conference around the chosen topic and be responsible for all organizational details. The new title of 'Conference'
would be applied since it suits better the distinctive character
which the annual meetings of ECCLS have assumed.

This year the title chosen for the seminar - Decentralized
Clinical Testing - had the same theme as that expressed in the
title of a newly formed standing action committee - Good Practices
in Decentralized Clinical Laboratories - chaired by Dr Dybkaer in
Copenhagen. This committee has seven subcommittees and it seemed
most appropriate that between them, with extra invited speakers,
they should run the conference as an expanded meeting of the
committees with participation from all registered attendees.

Contrary to the situation in previous seminars, Dr Dybkaer
was able to structure the presentations and debate, thus ensuring
optimal output, and the result was most rewarding in every way.
The presentations of Danish experts in various aspects were particularly appreciated.

FL Mitchell
ECCLS Chairman

List of Contributors

JE ASVALL
WHO Regional Office for Europe
8, Scherfigsvej
DK-2100 Copenhagen
Denmark

P BACKER
Institute for General Practice
University of Copenhagen
Juliane Maries Vej 18
DK-2100 Copenhagen
Denmark

DM BROWNING
Department of Clinical
  Chemistry
Wolfson Research Laboratories
Queen Elizabeth Medical Centre
Edgbaston
Birmingham B15 2TH
UK

DW DAWSON
Department of Haematology
North Manchester General
  Hospital
Manchester M8 6RB
UK

R DYBKAER
Department of Clinical
  Chemistry
Frederiksberg Hospital
Nordre Fasanvej 59
DK-2000 Frederiksberg
Denmark

R HAECKEL
Institut für
  Laboratoriumsmedizin
Zentralkrankenhaus
St Jürgen Strasse
D-2800 Bremen 1
FRG

RD JENNINGS
Department of Health and
  Social Security
Medical and Scientific
  Services Division
Hannibal House
Elephant and Castle
London SE1 6TE
UK

C KIRKEMO
Abbott Diagnostic Products
  GmbH
Max Planck Ring 2
D-6200 Wiesbaden-Delkenheim
FRG

LIST OF CONTRIBUTORS

H KÜFFER
Institut Central des Hôpitaux
  Valaisans
Division Chimie Clinique
CH-1951 Sion 3
Switzerland

D KUTTER
PO Box 748
L-2017 Luxembourg
Luxembourg

M LOCKER de BRUIJNE
Nursing Service
Hugo de Vriesweg 8
NL-9751PS Haren
The Netherlands

R NETTER
Laboratoire National de la
  Santé
25 Boulevard Saint Jacques
F-75014 Paris
France

P RIIS
Department of Medical
  Gastroenterology
Herlev University Hospital
Herlev Ringvej
DK-2730 Herlev
Denmark

RM ROWAN
Department of Haematology
Western Infirmary
Glasgow   G11 6TN
UK

E SIEDENFADEN
Vissinggaard
DK-8740 Braedstrup
Denmark

G SMART
Pathology Department
Southampton General Hospital
Tremona Road
Southampton   SO9 4XY
UK

N STORMBY
Division of Cytopathology
Malmö General Hospital
S-214 01 Malmö
Sweden

N TRYDING
Department of Clinical
  Chemistry
Central Hospital
S-291 85 Kristianstad
Sweden

CE WILDE
Department of Clinical
  Chemistry
Doncaster Royal Infirmary
Armthorpe Road
Doncaster   DN2 5LT
UK

Foreword

Decentralized clinical testing reaches back into antiquity as uroscopy, the scrutiny of urine and its sediments, then alchemy was applied by Philippus Aureolus Theophrastus Bombastus von Hohenheim alias Paracelsus (1493-1541), and later more specific procedures were introduced by Robert Boyle (1627-1691). The first clinical chemical laboratory was created in 1842 by Johann Joseph von Scherer in Würzburg, Germany, to reveal pathobiochemistry through more sophisticated analyses. Ward room and bedside testing, however, still thrived. The insatiable demand for clinical tests in ever-increasing numbers and varieties of quantities necessitated the birth, around the middle of this century, of the mastodontic, multipurpose and machine-cluttered central laboratory where the necessary expensive equipment and expertise could be utilized economically.

The pendulum is now swinging back towards analysis nearer the patient. There are three major reasons: (1) the increasing political emphasis on primary health services, (2) the timely monitoring of patients, and (3) the technical possibilities offered by analytical systems with an ingenious amalgamation of physics, electronics, chemistry and microprocessors, permitting selective analysis with inbuilt calibration and quality control. An awkward problem of this development is that the new equipment is often described as being problem-free for virtually any user after a minimum of instruction. Sometimes the claim is hedged by reassuring that screening results need not be as exact as those offered in a hospital by the central laboratory. This comforting viewpoint, however, is dangerous because the fate of a patient may well hinge on the primary result. As regards trouble-free operation, it remains an unobtainable ideal in spite of sophisticated engineering, and the detection of some malfunctions - not to mention repair - may require an experienced laboratorian rather than the casual physician or secretary.

It is unrealistic to expect every clinician to become a laboratory specialist, plowing through technical literature and checking performance claims for analytical systems. It is probably also not feasible to block the on-going deployment of vast numbers of decentralized analysers. The overriding consideration of any decentralizing process, then, is that it should only be implemented with a preliminary and running involvement of the expertise residing in the central laboratory. In general, the motto of the participants in this evolution - that is the decentralized user, the central clinical laboratory, the health service, industry, and the patient - should be cooperation and complement rather than combat. Only thus can the proper selection, procurement, maintenance and quality assurance of the analytical systems be ensured, resulting in relevance, quality and economy.

The managerial, educational, and economic problems involved are considerable and have already been debated during the last few years at dedicated meetings[1,2,3,4,5] - and at this ECCLS Conference. A number of articles have also appeared, and even a periodical[6], but a systematic treatise such as that for non-clinical laboratories[7,8] is not available.

Two bodies have now decided to address the special clinic test situation in a collaboration between health authority, industry, and the clinical laboratory professions. The National Committee for Clinical Laboratory Standards has created a task force on decentralized laboratories with working groups to cover different aspects of testing in the physician's office; already draft guidelines on some types of analytical systems and quality assurance are being circulated. The ECCLS has formed a Standing Action Committee on Good Practice in Decentralized Clinical Laboratories to examine testing in sites not managed by a central laboratory, i.e. ranging from the small hospital laboratory to the patient's home. During 1986 seven subcommittees have been formed to formulate guidelines on:

-       Reagents including reagent sets,
-       Quality requirements and quality assurance,
-       Premises and operational units,
-       Safety of personnel and environment,
-       Patient reception, preparation, and specimen handling,
-       Data flow and contacts, and
-       Management and organization.

Furthermore, liaison has been established with an ECCLS ad hoc committee on Good Clinical Laboratory Management and Practice.

The following pages present the views of different experts on the needs for decentralized testing, the available and future analytical systems, the cost implications, and the work problems of nursing and laboratory staffs. In a major section, ECCLS subcommittee spokesmen outline plans for their respective groups

FOREWORD

and present the issues to elicit comment.

It is the aim of these proceedings to show the health authority, the clinician and nursing staff, the manufacturer, and the laboratorian that adequate decentralized testing is a complex undertaking needing expert guidelines for non-experts - and that such guidelines are on their way.

René Dybkaer

REFERENCES

1. European Committee for Clinical Laboratory Standards (ECCLS), (1984). Gloag EA (ed.). Good manufacturing practice. Good clinical laboratory practice. The value of consultation between clinicians, surgeons and laboratory scientists. Proceedings of the 4th ECCLS seminar, Dublin.
2. Biomedical Business International (ed.), (1984). Clinical testing outside the hospital laboratory. A comprehensive one-day business seminar to help you take advantage of a rapidly growing clinical testing marketplace. (Biomedical Business International, Tustin) Washington.
3. Marks V and Alberti KGMM (eds.), (1985). Clinical biochemistry nearer the patient. Contemporary issues in clinical chemistry. Vol.2. (Churchill Livingstone, Edinburgh).
4. Hellsing K, Berg B, Jagenburg R, Kallner A and von Schenck H (eds.), (1986). Symposium on analytical systems near the patient, Uppsala. Upsala J Med Sci, 91, 119-227.
5. Appel W, (1986). Clinical biochemistry nearer the patient II. Mitt Dtsch Ges Klin Chem, 17, 183-187.
6. SPOT News (1985). Satellite and Physician's Office Testing: No 1 and following.
7. Department of Health, Education and Welfare (US), (1978). Food and Drug Administration. Nonclinical laboratory studies, good laboratory practice regulations (Final rule 1979-06-20). Fed Reg, 43, 59986-60025.
8. Organization for Economic Co-operation and Development (OECD), OECD principles of good laboratory practice. ENV/CHEM/MC/81.14,15-44.

Welcoming Address

It is indeed a pleasure for me to welcome this ECCLS conference here, the home of WHO's regional office for Europe. We have indeed cherished a longstanding cooperation with ECCLS and I am pleased to see among us today Dr Wahba, who for many years in his position as the responsible officer for EURO's activity within the field of laboratory technology ensured close contact with the ECCLS, and he continues to ensure this good cooperation today.

This meeting of the ECCLS comes at a particularly important time, and there are three reasons for this.

Firstly, we live today in an era of virtual scientific explosion, both in the field of medicine and in the many fields of science that contribute to the development of laboratory technologies. This has led to a rapid expansion in the laboratory sector - an expansion in the number of tests that can be offered to clinicians, a rise in the number and complexities of the apparatuses required by laboratories to follow these technological developments, and an increase in the demands made on laboratory staff for technical expertise as well as sheer workload.

This development has been very important in improving the possibilities for diagnosis and treatment in many areas of medicine and no one can doubt that we shall see a similar and perhaps even expanding trend, a quicker pace in development in the years ahead. This requires a professional body capable of supporting responsible developments internationally, and in my view the ECCLS has a very good potential for playing such a role.

Another reason why we are at a crossroads of development concerns current developments in thinking about health and health care. All who work in the health sector, or with health development issues, will have seen that during recent years we have witnessed an increasingly critical scrutiny by politicians, economists and even the public at large with regard to the sometimes marginal benefits of new investments in health care. Health care costs have reached a level where they cause serious debate and where quite drastic measures have been taken to curtail them in a rather summary fashion in many countries. There is simply a gradually growing feeling that perhaps not all new tests and not all new pieces of equipment may be cost/beneficial. In some instances this is also linked to questions of whether patient acceptability of new tests and procedures has always been sufficiently taken into account; at times patients may even feel that they are serving the equipment, and not the other way round.

The more fundamental issue of whether our national health policies are truly addressing the basic health problems, has recently been raised in a very serious fashion on a European level. Thus, from 1980 to 1984 the 32 countries of the WHO European Region - representing more than 800 million people, living in an area bordered by the Pacific Ocean coast of the Soviet Union in the east, the Mediterranean in the south and Greenland in the west - together developed a European health policy. It introduced fundamentally new priorities in health, inter alia, stressing the need to face, in a serious way, the problems of lifestyles, health and of better ensuring the appropriate use of technology in the health care system.

Finally, a third important factor of relevance to our meeting today is the steadily growing understanding - strongly emphasized in the new Regional Health for All Policy - that in today's Europe health development must be everybody's business: it must involve public as well as private initiatives; individuals as well as groups; institutions as well as public administrations. In this understanding the non-governmental organizations, in particular those representing the health professions, are increasingly recognized as key groups that must be intimately linked with the managing of future health developments. Thus, it is no coincidence that the technical discussions of the 1985 World Health Assembly concentrated on the role that non-governmental organizations have to play in the development of the Health for All Policy around the world, including also the European Region.

What are the implications of all this for the work of ECCLS? In my view, the development presents both a rare opportunity and a particular responsibility for ECCLS, a situation which the organization now should seriously consider. Up to now the organization has mainly concentrated on the problems of quality assurance in laboratory production processes. This certainly has been an important concern and no doubt the ECCLS should continue to be active in this field. However, in my view this is now far too narrow a scope: the real challenge is to move beyond quality assurance of laboratory procedures and to start looking also at the relevance, the usefulness and the cost/benefit analysis of laboratory tests in relation to their clinical use.

I am sure that there will be people in the audience who will frown on such a suggestion, saying that this can surely not be the responsibility of ECCLS, but that it is the responsibility and prerogative of the clinicians only. I would challenge them on that issue. Partly because clinicians themselves are not facing this serious problem squarely, and partly because I believe that laboratory professionals surely cannot agree to see themselves as the passive handmaidens of the clinicians only! They must share the responsibility for the clinical decisions that the use of their tests will entail and they must, in my view, accept the professional responsibility for initiating - when not already started - an active and continuous dialogue with their clinical colleagues on this issue. The laboratory specialists are the ones whose main interests lie with the laboratory tests, their use and production, and they must also be the ones with the main responsibility for assessing that these tests are not only reliable, but also used in the right way.

In my view, therefore, now is the time for the laboratory sector in general, and for ECCLS in particular, to start developing criteria for the appropriate use of laboratory tests, criteria that can lead to the establishment of appropriate information systems for monitoring and evaluating outcomes. Today we see far too much variation in the quantity and choice of clinical tests requested for similar clinical conditions from different practitioners and institutions, and this situation cannot be ethical in my view - neither vis-à-vis the patients who receive different types of care, nor with regard to society which does not have sufficient guarantee that the resources are used for the right priorities.

In this problem area we in WHO are extremely interested in developing a close cooperation with ECCLS. You will know that the Regional Office of WHO has for some time been developing programmes dealing with a broad range of appropriate technology issues, including also strong components related to the laboratory sector. We intend to push ahead in this area and I would like to use this occasion formally to extend to you an invitation to a joint ECCLS/WHO cooperation to develop criteria for the appropriate use of laboratory tests. Such criteria need to take into account not only safety, accuracy and effectiveness of laboratory tests, but also patient acceptability, health outcomes and cost/effectiveness of the use of such tests in practice. Such a cooperation should also include the development of appropriate information systems for routine use that can monitor these factors and provide for a constant feedback to individual laboratories and institutions of the quality of work that is performed. In this way each institution can learn from its own performance and compare with that of its colleagues in other institutions, as well as in other countries. This is the type of work where we will be willing to develop very concrete joint programmes with the ECCLS.

With this challenge to you I would, once again, like to welcome you to the Regional Office. I hope that your discussions will be both interesting and challenging and that the meeting can indeed mark a turning point for a more systematic cooperation between our two organizations on even more important issues in the future.

JE Asvall
Regional Director for Europe
World Health Organization

Part 1

WHAT IS THE NEED FOR DECENTRALIZED TESTING?

1
The Need for Decentralized Testing – A Patient's View

Eva Seidenfaden

I am a 35-year-old housewife, mother of three children (two of them three-year-old twins), a part-time teacher, and I am married to a doctor. I have had diabetes for six years and have tried six different insulin pumps but at present use the Novo-pen because my pump is out of order. I measure my blood sugar at least three times a day, and often more if I feel it necessary or want to try out a different treatment and change the amount of insulin. I use keto-sticks whenever the blood glucose is above 16-18 mmol/L and feel totally responsible for my own treatment. I regard the clinician and the general practitioner as my supporters and advisers.

My experiences lead me to conclude that home testing is absolutely necessary if a patient wishes to live a normal life, be responsible towards his or her illness and have the best treatment available.

ADVANTAGES OF HOME TESTING

Superior treatment

To have superior treatment requires having quick results in order to react to a specific blood sugar concentration. If one reacts quickly the chances of bad regulation are diminished and this leads to a feeling of physical well-being and psychologically one feels more secure. The knowledge of how to measure blood glucose and to act on the results provides an insight into the disease and into oneself. This is extremely valuable.

Traditional treatment where the patient goes to the clinic or to the general practitioner and gives a blood sample is, in my opinion, of little value. This is because the patient has either behaved differently prior to the examination in order to cheat, or is so upset that the result is misleading. Consequently this specific blood sample may lead to a change in the patient's treatment which may not be appropriate.

I therefore believe that being able to react wisely on the results of home testing is much better not only for the patient but also for the medical staff. The ability of the patient to understand or at least to describe his or her disease helps the clinical staff to advise in a much more meaningful way.

A sense of responsibility

Being able to treat oneself develops a very high sense of personal responsibility. No one else can be blamed when things go wrong and good regulation leads to feelings of pride and happiness. The results of home testing are always present and neglecting them would be very unwise. Although having to feel responsible can be psychologically difficult, I am sure the treatment is much more effective than that given only by professionals.

It is impossible - at least for me - to live on a tight time schedule and on a constant diet. It has always been very difficult for me to accept the facts of having to live a different lifestyle and of having a chronic disease with the constant fear of complications, and I find it hard to bear the feelings of guilt every time my diet is broken. The only way to accept these facts has been to understand the disease and to know how to treat it.

This kind of treatment demands special communication between the medical staff and the patient, and it must be discussed openly and in an atmosphere of understanding and mutual confidence. The medical staff probably know most about the disease in general, but the patient is certainly the one to know most about his or her feelings and have insight into the reactions of his or her disease. The patient must no longer be the silent, respectful and submissive person, and doctors must cease to be authoritarian and sometimes patronizing.

PROBLEMS WITH HOME TESTING

Psychological

Many psychological problems occur when the patient is expected to be responsible, and this must not be neglected. Human nature is fragile especially in those who are ill, and having a chronic disease may sometimes lead to a lack of courage. To be sensible and always react upon the signs of one's body or on figures on a display can be very discouraging and sometimes one feels like doing the opposite of all rules. Such neglect can be mortal, especially if one is not aware of the dangers. It is therefore very important that the information given by professionals is fully understood by the

4

patient and it is essential that the teaching provided is successful and competent.

The insulin pump, for example, is worn day and night and although one is aware of different bodily alarms and signs, difficulties can still arise in an awkward situation. For instance one might have flu, a high temperature, a husband away at work and three children screaming around the house - and then one has to measure the blood glucose. It is high - but is this because of the flu, the temperature, the children, the stress or what? In one such situation I had a slightly damaged pump tube which prevented the insulin from being injected and within a few hours I was acidotic, vomiting and very ill. Although I had monitored several times and kept on injecting insulin, it didn't occur to me until very late that my problem could be due to a lack of insulin. The pump showed no signs of deficiency. This example shows that although one tends to check everything it may be difficult to remember all possibilities.

Economic factors

In Denmark diabetics are paid 100 kr every 3 months to cover expenses. However my actual monthly expenses are as follows:

Diet	450 kr
Sticks	450 kr
Insulin	80 kr
Tubes and syringes	200 kr (approximately)
Total monthly expenses	1180 kr

Apart from 100 kr every 3 months these items are not subsidized. The investment in the necessary machinery is also an extra which must be met by the patient. This is unfair and creates unacceptable differences between people with different incomes. It seems that some companies even make considerable profit on home testing. For example, first they set an extremely high price on sticks and then invent a small expensive machine to cut the sticks in two!

Shortage of time

Time for testing may be a problem. Ideally it should of course be possible to find the time, especially when the importance of testing is considered. However, in everyday life factors such as stress, shyness and forgetfulness should not be forgotten. For instance when guests are coming for dinner there are a million things to prepare. Although my guests know about my diabetes, they don't think about it (luckily). Unfortunately in the middle of frying, baking, entertaining and laying the table it is far from convenient to measure blood sugar - which is quite ridiculous because it is precisely in this situation that it might be a good idea to change insulin delivery.

INCREASED DEMANDS ON THE HEALTH CARE SYSTEM RESULTING FROM GREATER PATIENT RESPONSIBILITY

Home testing has allowed me to have the best treatment available. In order to obtain it I have been a very active, inquisitive and sometimes a very annoying patient. I have never accepted anything but the very best equipment and have gone through the different aspects of the disease to a point that might have irritated the medical staff. My ambition has been to know everything, to act in a friendly way but never to accept being neglected. Such an attitude towards the medical system demands a certain character, a good backing from one's family and a strong feeling of self-confidence.

Not everyone has either the courage or such opportunities and therefore it is extremely important that the health care system helps the patient towards a deeper understanding of his condition. Being hospitalized puts a lot of people into a state of shock and they are not capable either of understanding and receiving all the facts and figures about the treatment, or of understanding the disease itself.

It is very important that the health care system provides different types of teaching, ensuring that the patient has got the idea of what it is all about. Teaching is not only words. Learning is feeling, touching, watching, hearing and having a direct contact with the teacher. It is important to have different teachers and members from all types of medical staff, and it is important that patients are able to exchange their views and experiences. Medical staff have often been working in an area of disease for several years and are therefore highly experienced and know everything worth knowing. But how much time do they actually spend with the individual patient - an hour, 5 minutes? Often the responsibility given to the patient is far bigger than the knowledge actually provided.

What is taught once is probably forgotten by the next lesson because all the terms and medical expressions are strange and unknown to the patient. A lot of repetition is necessary. I believe we all need a briefing once a year covering maintenance of the instruments, re-reading of manuals, discussion of treatment in special situations and a general talk about individuals' situations. Sometimes the responsibility is hard on the patient and can lead to feelings of guilt. Before it was much easier to say, 'My doctor says I may break rules once in a while'. This makes the patient feel happier and leaves the problem and the feeling of guilt to the doctor. Being responsible can be very tiring and I believe it should be a human right to be hospitalized or stay in another suitable place for a few days a year to take stock, to have an update on the main ideas about treatment and to have the chance of chatting, discussing and weeping with patients in similar situations. Leaving the responsibility to the patients means an enormous saving of money. The frequency of admissions will go down and I believe that the patients should be rewarded by having the right to a couple of days off from the responsibility.

THE IMPORTANCE OF CONSULTATION BETWEEN INSTRUMENT MANUFACTURERS AND THE PATIENT

The first year I wore a pump, daily I heard comments like 'What is that?', 'Do you really wear it 24 hours a day?' and, 'Isn't she too old to wear a Walkman!'. I felt that everyone's eyes were glued to the pump and all attention was given to the pump and not to me. I was almost envious! From the beginning I had chosen to personalize my pump. It was to become a 'she' and she was to become my very best friend. I would always be good to her and I would never quarrel with her. I know it sounds childish but after all the heavy discussions about treatment, handling the pump, insight into the disease and understanding consequences, and having used a lot of medical and theoretical terms, I felt the need to create my own little communication with the pump.

People's questions and the relationship between the pump and myself are two aspects of home testing that I think those dealing with treatment never think of. They consider only performance and although that is of course important it is essential that patients like the design of the instruments. They must be discrete, attractive to look at, made of good quality materials, and have an alarm that doesn't provoke divorce or wake the entire family in the middle of the night! When I was pregnant I often measured my blood sugar at night - sometimes several times. Having to measure at night seems hard enough - getting up to go to the bathroom and closing all the doors seems a punishment. Some of us (pregnant diabetics) tried to get the volume reduced and we succeeded with a number of machines. However this was only a limited victory since the majority of new machines have the same unacceptable high volume and tone. This example shows that when patients stand up for once and demonstrate, it helps - but only to a certain level. The producers of instruments should make contact with the patients on a much larger scale and discuss things such as design, sound stability and simplicity, and whether it can be dropped without breaking or is waterproof.

The language of the manual is very important and should be written by people who are experienced in teaching. Far too often the manuals are written by professionals who have neither insight into the disease nor the necessary psychological background, and do not use a vocabulary appropriate to formulating comprehensive texts.

It is appropriate to close with a quotation by Jan Carlzon, the managing director of Scandinavian Airlines. He says about responsibility, 'A person who is not informed cannot feel a responsibility. A person who is informed cannot avoid feeling responsible'.

Discussion

Boroviczény	How often do you use quality control?
Seidenfaden	Not as often as I should. The glucose meter should be checked once a fortnight but I do it once a year. I do not have it checked at the hospital but do take note of the colour on the strip and this gives me a rough guide to the accuracy of the instrument.

2

The Need for Decentralized Testing – A General Practitioner's View

Paul Backer

THE STIMULUS FOR CHANGE

The possibility of carrying out simple clinical tests and even more complex laboratory investigations in general practice has increased with changes in the organization of general practitioner services. For example the formation of multidisciplinary health centres or group practices with up to ten general practitioners encourages:

-   Greater professional contact between physicians with different interests including laboratory work;
-   Physicians to do more in general practice than single practitioners can do alone;
-   The establishment of better buildings and the pooling of resources; and
-   Regular participation in postgraduate education, research and teaching.

Laboratory tests carried out in general practice can now be paid for through health insurance and of course this will encourage more practitioners to consider carrying out tests locally. If more laboratory work could be carried out in general practice without increasing the total cost of laboratory tests, it would be in the interest of patients, society and doctors. Decentralized testing would:

-   Save time and money for the patients and society as a whole;
-   Reduce personnel costs in keeping these activities out of large institutions; and
-   Be more comfortable for the patient and satisfactory for the doctors.

THE PATIENT AND DECENTRALIZED TESTING

QUALITY REQUIREMENTS

If extensive laboratory testing is carried out in general practice, the quality must be equal to the quality in centralized laboratories. If this is not the case, the harm done to patients, society, the system and the reputation of the doctor will outweigh all the theoretical advantages.

If it is assumed that all laboratory tests relevant to general practitioners can be carried out in the health centre, the question of how much control is necessary must be addressed and how it can be done. It is possible roughly to divide clinical tests relevant to general practice into three groups:

(1)   Tests where no special control is necessary and the doctors only have to follow simple directions for use. These include tests done by sticks, tablets and powder and other simple examinations of urine and faeces.

(2)   Clinical tests, where the quality control can be carried out locally. There is a need for at least one responsible doctor with appropriate postgraduate education to take responsibility within the group. These tests include microscopic examinations of blood and urine, micro-organisms, skin temperature, audiometry, ECG, peak flow etc.

(3)   Clinical tests, where external expertise is necessary for the establishment of the laboratory, and for consultation and the performance of quality control procedures as in a centralized laboratory (e.g. electrolytes, hormones, enzymes, etc.). Furthermore, it must be mandatory for these tests to be carried out by trained laboratory workers.

If these conditions can be fulfilled, general practitioners in Denmark favour an extension of laboratory activity to their practices. If they cannot be met there is absolutely no interest in decentralization.

NEEDS AND RESOURCES

It must be emphasized that laboratory examinations are not a major part of the diagnostic work of the general practitioner. A maximum of 10% of all consultations lead to the performance of a laboratory test. Therefore a trained laboratory assistant can easily serve between 5-10 general practitioners with all the types of laboratory tests considered above.

In general, the needs for decentralized laboratory facilities are difficult to quantify because they depend on the organization of primary health care and on the individual doctor. In practices and systems where everything is paid for by society all of the above requirements for quality can be met and only the benefits to patients, society and doctors remain to be considered. In semi-socialized countries, like Denmark, where the physicians pay their own expenses and are free to do what they like, it can be said that need depends on the individuality and interests of the physicians and their attitudes to general practice.

All general practitioners wish to deal with illness as quickly as possible and the requirements of most patients, including emergency cases, will be covered by tests in groups (1) and (2) above. The most important reasons for establishing facilities for more complicated tests relate to geography and the interests of the doctor. Long travelling distances for the patients to centralized laboratory facilities motivates self-help in general practice.

CONCLUSIONS

In a system where the doctors themselves can decide what to do and how to do it, pure interest in doing even complex laboratory tests can lead to decentralization. However, the doctors must be aware of the demands of quality and quality control. In Denmark an acceptable position has probably been reached.

3

The Need for Decentralized Testing - A Hospital Clinician's View

Povl Riis

CONCEPTS

Decentralization presupposes the existence of a centre. This can be international, global or regional, or placed on the level of institutions, general practice or clinical departments. Clinical testing covers a number of specialities such as clinical physiology, clinical microbiology, clinical pathology, clinical imaging etc. In the present context clinical chemistry or clinical laboratory medicine is in focus.

THESES

The question of decentralizing clinical chemistry can be analysed in several ways:

(1) If the patient is the centre of all clinical activity (as many would without reservation claim), all so-called centralized systems are in fact decentralized.

(2) If clinical laboratory competence is situated far from the patient - as is often the case - the patient or material from the patient will have to be transported. If the patient or specimen cannot be transported, competence will instead have to be transported to the patient or be transferred permanently as part of a new administrative system.

(3) The relevance and the practicalities of bringing the patient (the clinical problem) and the clinical chemical competence in close contact depend on:

- Whether the analysis is a rare or a common procedure, the rare analyses being less suited for decentralization;

- Whether the analysis is simple or complicated, simple analyses often being common procedures, and rare analyses often being at the same time complicated ones;

- Whether the analysis is inexpensive or expensive, inexpensive analyses being mostly simple and common, and expensive ones generally being complicated and rare;

- Whether the level of service available varies with time (24 hours or weekly). For example few systems are able to compensate for a reduction in the availability of services during evenings, nights and weekends. Any system not able to compensate for such variability in service is of little use to clinicians and patients.

(4) Decentralization should never take place unless competent supervision can be guaranteed. This is almost the basic thesis of this matter.

(5) To improve the dialogue between clinical chemists and clinical decision-makers (i.e. consumers of clinical laboratory results) there should be attempts to introduce a simpler language. All too long we have suffered from Babylonic confusion because of terms such as accuracy and precision, which may be logical terms to use for teaching purposes but certainly do not facilitate daily dialogue. The ballistic analogies of placing shots close together but away from the target versus spreading them around a centre in or near the target ought to be substituted by simpler terms, such as the clincial quality of the test. This would presuppose a laboratory quality and cover within-sample and between-sample variation, coefficient of variation etc. We have a closely related analogue in the almost useless terms 'specificity' and 'sensitivity'. These are applied in the diagnostic context, often without the necessary adjectives, giving rise to huge transatlantic and inter-European confusions.

(6) Never centralize more unless the test service is still accessible close to the patient (or the clinical problem that she or he represents). Omit the adjective 'clinical' in clinical chemistry if such an accessibility does not exist.

(7) Centralization versus decentralization (whether the centre is defined in one way or the other) is not an either/or problem but a both/and problem, with the balance point as close to clinical chemical competence as possible, regarding clinical accessibility at the same time.

4

The Need for Decentralized Testing – A Laboratorian's View

Nils Tryding

THE CURRENT POSITION

New, quick and reliable techniques for laboratory analyses are now available for decentralized use in routine practice. However, before a decision is made to introduce these methods, discussion as to whether there is a need for them is necessary.

In southern Sweden, we have had regular contact between the laboratory and primary care doctors since the 1960s. We have registered which laboratory investigations are performed locally or sent on to the central hospital laboratory. Even more important are our regular meetings and discussions with clinicians on how to choose meaningful clinical chemical and haematological investigations in different clinical situations.

The physicians in primary health care have expressed three main wishes: They require:

(1) **Information** about test strategies and education of the personnel performing the laboratory tests;

(2) **Instrument servicing** for photometers, centrifuges and microscopes. In the beginning this service was badly needed. Some microscopes constantly showed the 'same' urine sediment picture.

(3) **Regular quality control** for the local analyses, especially blood haemoglobin. Documented good quality was preferred to quick but sometimes unreliable results.

We have made recommendations concerning choice of relevant laboratory tests for detection and follow-up of different diseases. These have also been discussed thoroughly in the Swedish Societies for Clinical Chemistry and General Practitioners as well as during twenty 5-day postgraduate courses for primary health care doctors and clinical chemists. A continuous re-evaluation is made.

THE ROLE OF THE CLINICAL CHEMISTRY DEPARTMENT

We have summarized the role of clinical chemistry especially in relation to decentralized testing in Table 4.1

Table 4.1 **The roles of the clinical chemistry department in decentralized testing**

---

(1)   Selection of analyses. The need for decentralized testing:
    (a)   Prevalence of disease
    (b)   Sensitivity and specificity of the method

(2)   Training

(3)   Selection of analytical technique

(4)   Quality assessment and guarantee

(5)   Information and education:
    (a)   Patient instructions
    (b)   Specimen collection and handling

(6)   Presentation and evaluation of results:
    (a)   Reference intervals and decision limits
    (b)   Effect of therapy

(7)   Responsibility according to law

(8)   Economic responsibility

Selection of tests

There are at least 32 reasons for requesting laboratory investigations[1]. Their meaningful use is highly dependent on the prevalence of the suspected disease. We must be aware of the fact that the prevalence of disease in primary health care is relatively low as compared to the situation in specialized university wards. When the prevalence is low the correct decision might even be not to perform a test. The clinical value of an assay is also of course dependent on the sensitivity and specificity of the method used.

After discussion with physicians in primary health care we have produced a detailed list of recommended analyses for use in the most common clinical situations. With respect to the techniques available today we have suggested which analyses can be performed locally and which should be sent to the hospital laboratory.

Almost all primary health care centres perform blood haemoglobin determination for which we have a well-organized quality control system in Sweden. The second most common laboratory investigation, erythrocyte sedimentation rate (ESR), has a long tradition. Patients do not feel they are thoroughly investigated unless an ESR is performed. The new vacuum technique for ESR determination has several advantages but still takes 60 minutes to perform and there is no quality control.

The clinical need for urine testing has been critically evaluated in Sweden. Routine investigation now includes only glucose and albumin determination. Other tests are performed only on suspicion of special diseases. In the recommendation of tests the most common diseases in primary care are included.

We have recently asked primary care doctors which laboratory tests they would like to have performed directly in their local clinics according to clinical needs. In addition to the tests already performed (blood haemoglobin, ESR, blood glucose, urine paper tests etc.) they also require plasma potassium and plasma creatinine. In our county the distance to hospital laboratories is short, but in other parts of Sweden where the distance is longer other tests might be added e.g. enzyme analyses for liver or heart disease.

New instruments are especially suitable for toxicological analyses and control of drug therapy. The need for this type of analysis was recently discussed and summarized at a joint meeting between the Swedish Society for Clinical Chemistry and the Centre for Toxicological Information, Stockholm[2]. The analyses which were felt to be of special value are listed in Table 4.2.

Table 4.2 Toxicology assays felt to be of special value

Necessary assays	Desirable assays
Paracetamol	Digoxin
Salicylate	Cholinesterase
Lithium	Theophylline
COHb	Isopropanol
Iron	
Ethanol	
Methanol	
Ethylene glycol	

The need for rapid answers is also well recognized in neonatal clinics. Serum bilirubin and C-reactive protein are examples of laboratory tests with high priority.

Training

There are special problems when instruments are used by untrained people. Even if an instrument is robust and functions well when used by trained laboratory personnel under optimal conditions, the performance can be very unsatisfactory when it is used by untrained staff. In primary health care there is a risk that many different untrained people will be involved. It may be necessary to issue some type of 'driver's licence' to achieve maximum security. Even after training some people may not be well suited to driving cars or new instruments!

Selection of techniques and quality assurance

As well as choosing the best analytical techniques documentation and guarantee of quality of analyses, is one of the clinical chemists' professional duties. The laboratory results obtained by the new techniques must be compared with standard routine analytical performance at the responsible hospital laboratory. If the same analyte concentration gives different results with different instruments there will be a risk of mistakes. This risk is obvious if the reference intervals for the same analyte differ in primary care using their special instrument and the central hospital using another instrument. Clinical chemical expertise is thus needed for harmonization and continuous control of analytical performance in primary health care as well as in hospitals. Quality assessment is a must. It includes continuous internal quality control as well as regular external quality registration. The term 'external quality control' should be avoided for psychological reasons. Great progress has been achieved by modern technology with increased analytical specificity and well controlled quality.

Information and education

In regular conferences with the clinicians who request tests we discuss which analyses can be recommended in different clinical situations. We also give training courses to staff performing the routine laboratory work in primary health care. In our experience this type of education is extremely important and very well received. Even in simple routine laboratory work the personnel involved need regular information in order to produce acceptable results with documented quality. The ideal situation seems to be that well-educated specialists in clinical chemistry be given the responsibility for education and quality assessment in a regional area.

The importance of biological variables must not be forgotten. The patient should be instructed to prepare appropriately before laboratory testing as this is sometimes necessary in order to get the correct result. All personnel involved in blood sampling must be aware of the necessity of using the correct technique. Thus muscle contractions in the arm during blood collection can falsely elevate the serum potassium values by up to 80%. Furthermore the correct handling of specimens is important, e.g. the separation of serum within 2 hours for potassium determination.

Presentation and evaluation of results

The clinical chemist must inform all users about actual reference intervals. Decision limits do not necessarily coincide with reference limits and should of course be related to each specific disease. Some analyses are specially well suited to follow-up of disease and control of the effect of therapy. As drugs are widely used we must also inform the users that drugs can alter laboratory test results, and not only because they have therapeutic effects. Drugs can also interfere with analytical determinations and they can have a great variety of biological effects. Literature references are collected and continuously evaluated in the Swedish drug information system[3].

New information has just become available concerning drug interference of results from new instruments used for analyses nearer the patient. The fact that some solid phase chemistry determinations are carried out on samples without dilution means that there is a greater chance of interference by drugs. The information is accessible via public telecommunication from a central computer or from the book 'Drug Interferences and Drug Effects in Clinical Chemistry'[3].

Economic considerations

Economy is an important factor with great impact on our work. Refunds given by insurance companies to hospitals or split between laboratories and wards are very important. Refund systems have resulted in great commercial successes for new techniques in some countries. In other countries where no refund is given, no single machine has been sold.

CONCLUSIONS

The great advantage of the new techniques is the offering of immediate answers when the physician and the patient are in personal contact. The laboratory test results can be evaluated immediately, together with other medical information. After further questions and investigations diagnostic decisions can be made without delay. The patients are saved travelling time and anxious waiting for answers. The nurses need not spend time on specimen handling for postal transport. The secretaries are saved clerical work. The physicians have the opportunity to make a final decision without extra communication by telephone or letter. Undoubtedly all types of people concerned are willing to pay well for this service. However, money is invested well only when the information obtained is reliable and clinically relevant.

REFERENCES

1.   Lundberg GD, (1983). Perseveration of laboratory test ordering: a syndrome affecting clinicians. J Am Med Assoc, 249, 639.
2.   Persson H, Hanson A and Tryding N, (1984). Behov av klinisk kemiska undersökningar finns vid akuta förgiftningar. Läkartidningen, 81, 1321-1322
3.   Tryding N and Roos K-A, (1986). Drug Interferences and Drug Effects in Clinical Chemistry. 4th Ed.(Stockholm: Apoteksbolaget)

Discussion

Bonini   Sometimes it will be necessary for the patient to return to the doctors office so that a sample can be obtained at the correct time and the potential advantage of having decentralized testing available will be lost.

Tryding   Perhaps circadian rhythms should be taken into account more in deriving reference ranges.

Part 2

WHAT IS BEING PROVIDED BY INDUSTRY FOR DECENTRALIZED TESTING?

5

Equipment for the Side Ward, the Doctor's Premises and the Patient's Home

Curtis Kirkemo

INTRODUCTION

The health care industry is undergoing considerable changes today. These changes are being driven by four sources: technologists, government and related reimbursement issues, health care providers and health care users. The principal causes of these changes are advances in technology, cost containment, changing demographics of doctors and patients, lower interest rates making equipment more affordable, increased competition for patients and demands for service from patients and families.

INDUSTRY'S RESPONSE TO CHANGE

To understand industry's response to the changes, one must consider two general concepts.

The first of these is the concept of the S-curve. The theory states that for any endeavour the relationship between effort and benefit is an S-shaped curve. Initially a large effort is required to see significant benefit, followed by a large increase in benefit per unit effort, and then again tapering off to smaller benefits per unit effort. In technology, this translates into a situation where any technology will become old and no longer return the significant financial benefits which would justify continued research investments. At that point it is necessary to move to a newer technology and with it to a new S-curve in order to continue to achieve a desired benefit to cost ratio. The impact of this is that there is always going to be a major effort on the part of any company to make the jump to a new S-curve before its competitors do.

The second concept is that of movement of technology closer to the end user. The example which best displays this is the computer industry. The technology for making computers was initially very expensive and consequently computers were largely owned by well-financed users with the capital to afford them. The average user would then rent time on the machines. As the market has matured the computer industry has sought continued growth by making computers simpler to use and less expensive, a development from which the industry can profit via large sales volumes. As we have seen in recent years this has reached the point where many homes now have personal computers. The same pressures and opportunities are driving the diagnostics industry to develop products for decentralized users.

Both of these concepts are useful for understanding the natural progression of technical advancement. The challenge for those of us working in the health care field is to find ways of most smoothly incorporating, accepting and beneficially controlling these changes.

REQUIREMENTS FOR USERS OF DECENTRALIZED TESTS

Are the requirements of decentralized users of diagnostic tests different from those of traditional users? In many ways they are not but there are certain characteristics which are needed to make decentralized testing more useful:

- **Ease of use** is important since a decentralized facility will not necessarily have highly trained staff. This will certainly be true for home testing.

- The system will need to be **labour saving**. Labour is the largest controllable cost in testing, and systems which require more labour than current systems will certainly not be widely adopted.

- The results will have to be **reliable,** ideally more so than current tests.

- The systems will need to have **good versatility**. If instrumentation is required then it is important to have versatility in order to benefit maximally from capital and space investment.

- Many alternate site testing facilities are space limited and therefore **size of the equipment** is another important issue.

- Finally it will be necessary to provide **good service** at a **reasonable cost**.

Quality control of alternate site testing is another issue which must be considered. Regardless of where the testing is done, there are four aspects which need to be controlled. These relate to test **sensitivity, specificity, reproducibility** and **reliability**.

Table 5.1 Strengths and weaknesses of five different analytical systems suitable for decentralized clinical chemistry testing

Strengths	Weaknesses	Strengths	Weaknesses
Ames Seralyser		**Dupont ACA IV**	
Low cost	Serum only	Easy to use	High cost
First on the market	Requires precision pipetting	No pipetting	Serum only
Reasonable test menu	Requires dilutions	Large test menu	90-day warranty
Acceptable warranty	Requires changing modules	Walk-away capability	Large size
	No walk-away capability	Printout	Separate electrolyte unit
	No printout	Random access	Disposables, buffers, waste
	No random access	Excellent throughput	Requires storage space
	No sodium test	Hotline	
Kodak DT-60		**Abbott Vision**	
Relatively low cost	Serum only	Whole blood	Moderate menu
Compact	Requires precision pipetting	Easy to use	Moderate cost
Walk-away capability	Limited test menu	No pipetting	
Printout	Freeze/thaw slides	Random access	
Random access	Separate electrolyte and enzyme modules at extra cost	Immunoassays	
Fast throughout	No immunoassays	Electrolytes	
		Compact	
		Walk-away capability	
		Printout	
		Simple calibration	
		Moderate menu	
		Good throughout	
		Good warranty	
		Hotline for questions	
Boehringer Mannheim Reflotron			
Whole blood	Limited test menu		
Moderate cost	Precision pipetting		
Self-calibrates	No electrolyte tests		
Acceptable warranty	Requires changing modules		
	No walk-away capability		
	No printout		
	No random access		

AVAILABLE INSTRUMENTATION

Today industry is making products for three principal types of alternate use. They are for critical care facilities, for the physician's office and to a limited extent for the home.

Critical care testing largely concerns blood gases, electrolytes, and selected metabolites (e.g. pregnancy screening). The physician's office testing historically covers the following areas: multiparameter urine dipsticks, haematology, clinical chemistry and immunoassays.

The instruments of major interest to this conference are those designed to do clinical chemistry measurements. This is the area undergoing the most rapid change today in terms of where the testing can be done. There are five primary systems being offered for the critical care and physician's office areas. They are the Ames Seralyzer, the Kodak DT-60, the Dupont ACA IV, the Boehringer Mannheim Reflotron and the Abbott Vision. Table 5.1 lists some of their strengths and weaknesses.

These indicate that the current state of technical development is allowing testing to be run in non-traditional sites, but also that we are not at a state of technical development which is ideal yet. The Vision is an example of what the best current technology will allow us to do. In this instrument the tests are carried out in disposable plastic cartridges, about 6 cm x 5 cm, which are barcoded for instrument reading. The sample is whole blood either from a normal tube drawing or from a fingerstick. It is added to the test cartridge either by adding a drop of blood to the well on top of the cartridge or by drawing the blood into a capillary and inserting the capillary into the cartridge. No precision measurement is required. The cartridge is next inserted into the instrument and it is designed to fit only one way into the machine. Finally, after closing the instrument door, the button labelled 'Run' is pressed. The instrument reads the various assays that are present, runs and then gives the determined values for the samples as a paper printout. Ten samples can be run at one time in random order. Quality control is maintained by use of traditional calibrators and controls. A control should be run daily for each assay and the instrument recalibrated when the controls indicate the need.

NON-INSTRUMENTAL SYSTEMS

Non-instrumental systems available today fall into four basic types. The standard dry chemistry dipsticks which were introduced by Ames in the 1940s are available for many urine tests as well as some blood chemistries. Agglutination tests have been sold for 10-15 years now with home pregnancy tests being the most familiar. Recent years have seen the development of EIA's for this market. These come in many formats, but are basically the traditional EIA assay systems developed to be easier to run and to be read by eye. A final approach that should be mentioned briefly is the marriage of the biology of assays with electronics in what can be grouped together under the name 'biosensors'. These are small electrical devices whose electrical output is modulated by a biological component in serum or urine. We are just beginning to see examples of these reach the market.

What types of tests are being done with these systems? Most physicians are using some form of the dipstick for basic urine testing. It is in the home market where there is a growing use of this type of testing. The principal current usages are in diabetic monitoring, pregnancy testing, faecal occult blood testing and the recent use of home testing for ovulation prediction. Future likely candidates for home testing are Strep-A, UTI, STDs and AIDS. Because of the wide variety of non-instrumental systems available it is not possible to consider all approaches. However, the Abbott Testpack system which is a recent entry into this area may be used to illustrate the current state of the art.

The Testpack is basically a reformatting of the standard sandwich EIA into a system which is faster and easier to run. For HCG, five drops of urine are added to the filter and allowed to be absorbed. Next three drops of reagent A are added and allowed to soak in for 1 minute. The filter is removed and approximately 1 mL of reagent B is added. After the solution has been absorbed three drops of reagent C are added and allowed to react for 2 minutes. About 1 mL of reagent D can be added at this time to stop the reaction and the answer is read. The total time for this assay is about 5 minutes. The answer is positive (50 IU cutoff) if a positive (+) sign shows on the Testpack and negative if a negative sign (-) shows. The important point here is that the negative indicator is built into the system to assure that the test was run with the correct protocol. If an improper protocol was used there would be no reading on the Testpack and the operator would be instructed to run another test after studying the protocol. The speed and reproducibility of this type of system make it possible to consider doing just about any standard immunoassay by this method. The system is certainly simple enough at this point for a person with minimal training to operate and is therefore easily applied to physician's office testing. With further simplification this type of technology will be useful as a home diagnostic.

LOOKING TO THE FUTURE

An assay system is composed of multiple technologies. For most immunoassays these can be thought of as the following: a selective probe, a signal generator, a solid phase, and a formating scheme. Each of these areas is undergoing very rapid change. Monoclonal antibodies are just beginning to make major changes in what can be done in assays. Their potential will continue to be rapidly developed. The use of DNA probes is the next major change in probe technology and will have a significant impact on testing within the next 5 to 8 years. Breakthroughs have been made in both instruments and chemistry for reading signals such as time-resolved fluorescence and chemiluminescence. The added stability and sensitivity of these methods and others will enable industry to develop systems with unique characteristics. Finally major breakthroughs in the characteristics of solid phases will enable the design of faster and simpler systems with accuracy and reliability that will surpass our current best standards. As an indication of what may result Figure 5.1 shows the basic outline of a complete instrument on a single silicon chip. This includes the ability to run the biological part of the assay on a small chip with all the electronics, sample handling and optics built into the chip. This type of system may not be available in the immediate future but the fact that it can be designed on paper is an indication that the appropriate technologies are being developed.

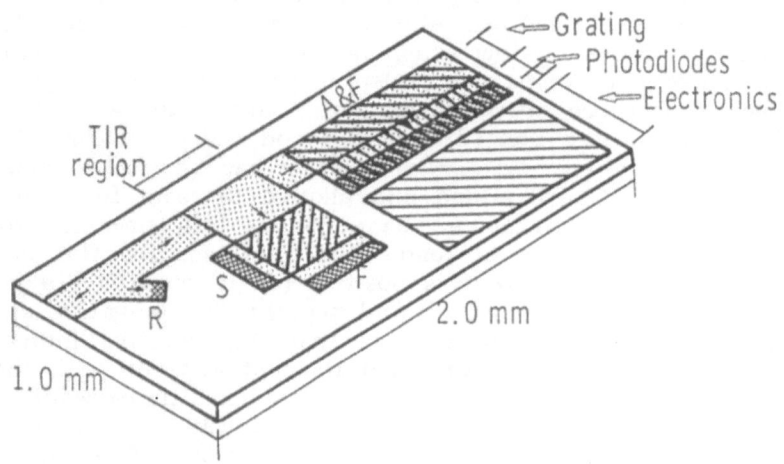

Figure 5.1 Instrument on a chip.

TIR = Total Internal Reflection; R = Reference; S = Scattering;
A = Absorbance and Fluorescence; F = Fluorescence

CONCLUSIONS

In view of the rapid change that new technology will bring, it is important to conclude with some comments on how to control the changes. In seeking ways to develop standards and regulations controlling future technologies it is necessary to think not only in terms of the traditional testing sites and related problems but instead to view these changes from a technological perspective. Specifically new assays should be assessed by the following characteristics:

EQUIPMENT FOR DECENTRALIZED TESTING

- What is the reliability of the procedure?

- What degree of personal judgement is required to run the assay?

- What personal skills are needed?

Standards and regulations must be supportive of technical advancement and flexible enough to apply to probable future technologies.

Part 3

IS THE CHANGED RESPONSIBILITY WELCOME?

6

Is the Changed Responsibility Welcome? A Nurse's View

Margreeth Locker de Bruijne

INTRODUCTION

Everyone involved in patient care wishes to arrive at the correct diagnosis as quickly and with as few investigations as possible so that appropriate therapy can be rapidly introduced and the patient restored to health. The laboratory is very important in the diagnostic process and a wide variety of tests may be carried out depending on the clinical situation.

Advances in technology now permit an increasing number of tests to be performed outside the central laboratory. From the nurse's point of view these developments have both advantages and disadvantages which are considered below.

ADVANTAGES OF DECENTRALIZED TESTING

Theoretically there are considerable advantages to be gained if modern analytical and computer techniques can be harnessed to enable nursing staff to produce reliable test results. These include:

(1) 24 h availability of tests;
(2) Minimal delay in the case of emergencies;
(3) No problems with misplaced samples and results;
(4) No rushing to the central laboratory outside normal laboratory hours;
(5) No need to call out the duty analyst at night.

In addition, the organization and dispatch of samples to the central laboratory and the filing of all results can take an enormous amount of time for the nursing staff and their administrative assistants. Some of these problems would be minimized with the availability of testing facilities on the ward.

DISADVANTAGES OF DECENTRALIZED TESTING

There are of course disadvantages and problems with decentralization:

(1)   Tests which are the basis for diagnosis and therapy must be absolutely reliable;
(2)   The total number of tests performed is often very large;
(3)   The types of tests are very varied;
(4)   The performance of the tests takes time;
(5)   Test results are the responsibility of clinical chemists.

When one thinks of the need for a decentralized laboratory service it is necessary to distinguish between the routine tests and those required for the immediate management of the patient. In view of the large number and wide variety of routine investigations most nurses would prefer this testing to be performed in a large central laboratory.

REQUIREMENTS FOR DECENTRALIZED TECHNIQUES

When a decentralized technique becomes available it should fulfil the following requirements:

(1)   It must be reliable;
(2)   It must be rapid to perform;
(3)   It should use equipment which is easy to handle;
(4)   The equipment must not need cleaning after every test;
(5)   The results should preferably be presented on a printout;
(6)   It should be easy to learn to use the equipment with the help of simple instructions.

LOOKING TO THE FUTURE

In these days of intensive automation and computerization it must be possible to have in the central laboratory a computer which is connected to all terminals on the wards. As soon as the analysis is completed, it should then be possible to view the data on the ward terminal simply by keying in the patient code. Such systems are now becoming available in some American hospitals and they reduce considerably the need for any decentralization of laboratory services.

CONCLUSIONS

Nurses on general wards, outpatients departments and intensive care units will welcome decentralized laboratory services for emergency tests in the evening, during the night and over the weekend. However, the bulk of complicated analyses must be performed by professional people in a central laboratory which is within walking distance of the wards and ideally the results should be available on ward terminals.

7

Is the Changed Responsibility Welcome? A Laboratorian's View

Graham Smart

GROWTH OF DECENTRALIZED TESTING

Decentralized testing is not new. There is ample evidence that decentralized testing takes place in intensive care units, coronary care units and special care baby units. Browning et al.[1] published a survey of clinical chemistry equipment outside central laboratories and highlighted the problems faced with the ad hoc purchase of testing equipment outside the laboratory. These are a lack of recognition that the instrumentation requires day-to-day maintenance and servicing, that the instrumentation requires basic skills for its accurate operation, and that it also requires the application of quality control procedures.

Reasons for the establishment of these decentralized testing facilities are difficult to ascertain and we can only guess at them. However, they do not appear to have been established following a detailed consideration, involving the local laboratory, of the perceived needs of the purchasers. This seems to have been avoided because the equipment has been bought from private or research funds. The facilities are frequently not welcomed by the central laboratory, particularly when the first indication the laboratory has of the existence of a decentralized testing facility is the comments of a clinician that the laboratory's results do not correlate with those which he has himself achieved.

This way of establishing decentralized testing facilities in no way changes the responsibilities of the laboratory inasmuch as the laboratory cannot be held responsible for such facilities, not having been involved in the initial decision-making process which established them. The ad hoc arrangement outlined here is only one way in which decentralized testing facilities can be established. However, it may well be the way that decentralized testing will be established outside hospitals, i.e. in general practitioner practices and health centres. It should not be the way that decentralized testing starts within hospitals.

REGULATION OF DECENTRALIZED TESTING

Within hospitals procedures should be formulated such that requests to carry out testing outside the central laboratory must be evaluated, taking account of the implications to the laboratory and to the hospital itself. The first step in such a procedure would be to place an embargo on the purchase of analytical equipment outside laboratories without first having sought the advice of the laboratory. This would mean that clinicians wishing to establish out-of-laboratory testing would be required to produce a case of need which could then be examined and costed. This exercise should examine other ways, including centralized testing, of meeting the needs of the clinicians concerned. The implications to the laboratory of such an alteration should also be identified. If the examination of the proposal shows that there is a justifiable need to set up out-of-laboratory testing then the laboratory should be involved in advising the clinician what type of instrumentation to buy. This would involve carrying out an evaluation to show that the instrument would meet the proposed needs and be capable of being used in its decentralized location.

Additional responsiblities which would fall on the laboratory would be the training of staff who are likely to use the instrumentation, its maintenance on a day-to-day basis, the establishment of quality control procedures and educating the users regarding health and safety needs in handling specimens. The resource implications of these activities must be taken into account in arriving at a final conclusion. If it is decided to establish a decentralized testing facility it should then become the laboratory's responsiblity to establish quality control and quality assurance procedures and to monitor via these procedures the usage of the equipment and the competence of its users. Regular attempts should be made to re-evaluate the original purchasing decision and to identify extra training and/or educational needs of the staff using it.

This type of structured approach to the establishment of out-of-laboratory testing puts changed responsibilities on the laboratory, and contrasts sharply with the ad hoc method of establishing out-of-laboratory testing which puts no responsibilities on the central laboratory. In the latter situation the laboratory cannot be held responsible for decisions over which it had no control and the responsibility lies very clearly with the purchaser and the supplying manufacturer. However, the structured approach to the purchase of testing equipment within hospitals is equally applicable to large health centres and general practitioner practices. There is no particular reason why they need to make their purchases on an ad hoc basis and it would be better for their practice and for the patients if they were to consult laboratories at least on the suitability of the instrumentation they intend to purchase.

CHANGING RESPONSIBILITIES

The system outlined above would certainly put changed responsibilities on the laboratory. Whether these responsibilities were welcome or not would depend upon the effect decentralized testing had on the central laboratory. The possible effects are that it would produce either less or more work, or leave the workload unchanged. If decentralized testing produced less work by removing from the laboratory normal and unnecessary requests then this would leave the laboratory more time to devote its attentions and its scarce resources to those investigations requiring specific and detailed work-up and, in consequence, the changed responsibilities brought about by decentralized testing would be welcomed within the laboratories. If it produced more work, as could be the case if the equipment or the user produced wrong results, then the increased demand upon the laboratory in correcting the results and re-educating the users would not be welcomed. Also, from the user's point of view, the credibility of the equipment would rapidly diminish and one could be faced with comparatively expensive equipment lying idle in wards and side rooms. If the workload remained unchanged, laboratories would not welcome the increased responsibilities put on them in terms of advice on purchasing and maintenance, training and the establishment of quality control, as these would require extra resources within the laboratory and the cost/effectiveness of decentralized testing procedures would then have to be challenged.

CONCLUSIONS

If sensible procedures of the type outlined above are used to evaluate and establish decentralized testing, then the changed responsibilities facing the laboratory will be welcomed and accepted. If, however, purchase of such equipment takes place without consultation with the laboratory and attempts are later made to make the laboratory responsible for the outcomes of these systems, this extra responsibility will be resented by laboratories.

REFERENCES

1.   Browning DM, Cowell DC, Kilshaw D, Knowles D, Randall J and Singer R, (1984). Clinical chemistry equipment outside laboratories. Med Lab Sci, 41, 99-107.

Discussion

Kirkemo	Are there any obstacles other than human nature which prevent clinical chemists taking an active role in introducing decentralized instruments?
Smart	No
Dybkaer	Problems often exist when a clinician has his own laboratory and is reluctant to give it up.
Landaas	Ideally central laboratories should select equipment and be responsible for education. In Norway we are trying to make this approach work.

Part 4

THE ROLE OF ECCLS IN STANDARDS FOR GOOD PRACTICE IN DECENTRALIZED CLINICAL LABORATORIES

8

Premises and Operational Units

David Browning

INTRODUCTION

A recent tragedy in the UK highlighted once again the need for careful assessment of the requirements for laboratory services to patients. In this particular tragedy a mistake at the bedside of an unconscious patient was compounded by an incorrect result being given by a glucose analyser in the laboratory. The biochemist in charge of the laboratory said that a study in Glasgow had demonstrated that as many as one in ten of 'BM-strip' tests give inaccurate results because nurses do not follow the instructions properly. At the end of the inquest the coroner recommended a more rigorous training programme for nurses using such equipment outside the laboratory.

QUALITY OF WORK IN DECENTRALIZED LABORATORIES

The present situation

There is good reason to believe that the standard of work produced by decentralized laboratories or by units using equipment at the bedside and away from the conventional laboratory is less good than it should be when compared with results from conventional laboratories. Table 8.1 shows the results from a recent national survey in the UK. A quality control specimen, reconstituted and routed through conventional laboratories but analysed outside laboratories by non-laboratory personnel, shows clearly that the imprecision of results from non-laboratory workers is greater than that from conventional laboratories. The results from those carrying out glucose determinations are particularly worrying. In addition the results from those using dipsticks and visual readings ranged from 2.2 to 44.0 mmol/L. Since this survey was routed through the central laboratories it can be assumed that these results are from those hospitals where there is a measure of cooperation between the main laboratory and the 'decentralized laboratory'.

Table 8.1 Extra-laboratory equipment (second survey)

Test	n	mean	SD	CV	Lowest	Highest	Range
Sodium (mmol/L)							
NEQAS	412	151.25	1.82	1.2	141	165	24
Extra-lab	69	152.8	2.4	1.6	146	166	20
Potassium (mmol/L)							
NEQAS	422	6.15	0.12	1.9	4.5	7.8	3.3
Extra-lab	71	6.17	0.19	3.0	4.7	7.2	2.5
Glucose (mmol/L)							
NEQAS	418	13.40	0.48	3.6	6.2	16.09	9.89
Extra-lab	492	13.60	1.98	14.6	1.5	22.0	20.5

Values shown represent overall results after exclusion of results outside two standard deviations. NEQAS (National External Quality Assessment Scheme) results were obtained in central laboratories.

Future expectations

Equipment outside laboratories is not a new phenomenon but in a survey carried out in the UK in 1984[1] it was shown that there was active cooperation between the central laboratory and the ward or clinical unit carrying out the tests in less than 50% of the 210 who replied to a questionnaire.
      There can be little doubt that results produced on equipment closer to the patient are more convenient and faster, and allow decisions on diagnosis and treatment to be made much more quickly. It is however quite unreasonable that lower standards of results should be tolerated in these circumstances. It can be argued that less inaccuracy and imprecision will be required since these results will be acted upon immediately by the clinical staff. It is known that contributory factors to producing high quality data are environment and facilities, and it is essential that the standards expected of a clinical laboratory should also apply to **premises** and **operational units** or decentralized laboratories where the vital work will be carried out. There is the alternative that we accept a lower quality of test result information from decentralized laboratories, but in view of the effort which has gone and continues to go into producing high quality data from laboratories it is doubtful if many laboratory workers would find that concept acceptable.

STANDARDS FOR PREMISES AND OPERATIONAL UNITS

One of the many problems of decentralized laboratories is that they are inevitably smaller than conventional laboratories but are multi-disciplinary, the range of tests and the facilities required thus being wide (Table 8.2). The standard of facilities available must obviously reflect the type of work to be carried out and these standards will be different in intensive therapy units, in a hospital or in a general physician's office. Regulations regarding standards will also be easier when there are managerial and administrative links with conventional laboratories. As technology advances, so will the demands for more monitoring of treatment in the patient's home, and it would seem unreasonable to demand laboratory facilities in a patient's home where glucose determinations only are to be performed.

Table 8.2 Possible sites for decentralized testing

---

1. In hospitals where there is a conventional clinical laboratory but a physician, for many reasons, may wish to arrange for tests to be done closer to the patient (intensive therapy unit, renal unit, special care baby clinic or a ward laboratory for a specialist group of patients).
   No administrative or managerial link to the laboratory.

2. In an out-patient or casualty department.
   No link to the laboratory.

3. Private hospitals.
   Small multidisciplinary laboratories often with no medical or senior scientist consultant cover.

4. Physician's or general practitioner's office, group practice or clinic.
   No conventional laboratory. No trained staff.

5. Clinical side rooms in hospitals.
   No link with the laboratory.

6. At the bedside.

7. In the patient's home for self-monitoring or routine treatment.

In the final analysis, however, the motives for introducing standards in premises and operational units must be to safeguard and preserve the standard of patient care, and regulations introduced for self-interest, perfectionist or professional protection reasons will be doomed to failure. It is easy to conceive regulations which will apply to laboratories where a single or perhaps two analysers related to the same discipline will be installed but these will be increasingly unlikely situations in the future. A major difficulty facing those formulating regulations is the diversity of ac-

45

tivity and range of places in which they will be found. These are so wide and range from the intensive therapy unit in a hospital to a general practitioner's office. Technology has advanced so that it is possible to carry out an impressive range of tests in several disciplines of pathology on equipment which is becoming increasingly simple to use. The problems that laboratories have faced will now have to be faced by decentralized laboratories. The days when health care workers and laboratory scientists were expected to work in slums, with all the attendant dangers, are long gone. Recommendations on premises must address themselves to the following:

- Risks of infection and ease of decontamination;
- Space and shape (these units are rarely purpose-built);
- Type of equipment;
- The necessary mix of equipment;
- The availability of general laboratory supplies;
- Wall, ceiling and floor surfaces;
- Windows, light and sun in relation to equipment;
- Air exhaust, ventilation and air conditioning;
- Washing facilities and the possible need for showers;
- Electrical outlets;
- Benching - surfaces, sealing, heights;
- General furnishings and storage;
- Telephone; and
- General decor - lighting and colours.

CONCLUSIONS

Staff unfamiliar with laboratory procedures must not be exposed to unnecessary risks as a result of poor facilities, and the setting up of decentralized units must be such that they will be conducive to good environmental standards and high quality work. The subcommittee on premises and operational units is addressing itself to these and other problems and it is inevitable that some overlap of our deliberations with those of other subcommittees will occur. What will remain uppermost in our subcommittee's deliberations is that the quality of test results and ultimately the service to the patient must not be allowed to deteriorate.

REFERENCES

1. Browning DM, Cowell DC, Kilshaw D, Knowles D, Randall J and Singer R, (1984). Clinical chemistry equipment outside laboratories. Med Lab Sci, 41, 99-107

Discussion

Boroviczény   It is important to have an ECCLS standard for rooms where equipment is to be used both in a centralized and decentralized situation. I do not know of any.

Browning   In the UK there are national standards for main laboratories.

Dybkaer   The ECCLS already has an ad hoc committee on good laboratory practice chaired by Professor Leijnse. In the standing action committee on good practice in decentralized clinical laboratories we must concern ourselves with work in decentralized laboratories.

Hjelm   Dr Browning asked who should be responsible for advising patients at home. I believe that the central laboratory should do this since instruments such as glucose meters fail on many occasions because instructions are poorly given by clinicians.

Browning   I would take that one further. The patient should actually visit the laboratory and have his instrument checked periodically.

Dybkaer   All such instruments should be linked into some type of quality assurance system.

Netter   What about pregnancy testing?

Browning   I don't think that this sort of test should be available for patients to use themselves.

9

Methods and Reagents

Hans Küffer

INTRODUCTION

Decentralized clinical laboratory testing is expanding more and more, mainly in the fields of haematology, microbiology and clinical chemistry. In this paper special attention is given to clinical chemistry. However most of the remarks and recommendations will also be applicable to other laboratory disciplines.

Decentralized clinical laboratory testing in the hospital may be considered for the following areas:

- emergency admissions,
- intensive care,
- surgery,
- resuscitation units,
- dialysis,
- paediatrics, and
- the night doctor's office.

METHODS

Each method employed in a diagnostic laboratory procedure comprises all the components going into the production of the final reported result: procedure, materials, equipment and personnel. Thus an analytical procedure proposed for use in a decentralized laboratory should sufficiently define each determinant of the final result such that operation within the tolerances specified ensures performance within the limits claimed[1].

49

Test selection

Test selection for decentralized testing in the hospital should be made by the central laboratory manager using the same care as indicated in 'Guidelines for Kit Evaluation'[2].

Decentralization of clinical laboratory procedures should be considered only if the following conditions are fulfilled:

(1)   Clinical usefulness:
-    Immediate response is necessary (e.g. glucose);
-    The sample may alter during transportation (e.g. urine leukocytes[3].

(2)   Practicability:
-    The methodological basis guarantees performance within the limits claimed;
-    The method is robust, and thus alterations during handling and change of environment have a tolerable effect or none at all on the quality of the analytical output;
-    The documentation of results, quality control and logs is guaranteed.

(3)   Cost-effectiveness:
-    The cost of external laboratory testing should be less than or equal to classical laboratory procedures. If the clinical usefulness is fulfilled, the effectiveness will increase.
-    Since most reagent sets are much more expensive than the methods fully installed in a central laboratory, the argument of needing immediate results has to be checked carefully. The problem may be solved more economically by improving the data-processing rather than by decentralizing the analytical work. The turnaround time is an important analytical goal to be defined for each test discussed for decentralization.
-    If by decentralization of clinical laboratory testing the stat-laboratory can be omitted, a considerable economy is possible.

Techniques

The simplified techniques used in decentralized laboratories may be qualitative, semi-quantitative or quantitative procedures. The qualitative and semi-quantitative techniques involve the greatest problems, since they involve measurements of a continuum for which discriminative limits must be established[1].

(1)   Directly readable results: Turbidity and visual change of

colour is widely used for qualitative pregnancy and drug abuse testing. The results depend considerably on the person performing the reading, especially at borderline values. Training and experience are therefore imperative. These tests must not be used in occasional testing.

(2)   Reflectometry: Semi-quantitative and quantitative testing by 'dry chemistry' or dipsticks may be evaluated by visual colour change and comparison with a colour-scale or by instrumental measurement or reflectance.

(3)   Photometry: Beside the euphoric development in 'dry chemistry', classical 'wet chemistry' in prepacked form nowadays covers a broad test programme. Easy to use, these tests may take the fancy of untrained people. However, if the tests are performed by an operator with limited analytical knowledge, he must be supervised by trained staff.

(4)   Electrodes: Electrodes are most widely used for the determination of blood gas and electrolytes.

Performance claims

(1)   Turnaround time: For glucose and potassium, the total time which elapses between the clinician taking the specimen and the laboratory reporting the results should be 30 min or less. For urea, haemoglobin and CSF and urine analyses, the turnaround times should be 60 min or less and, for other analyses, in emergency situations, 120 min or less is reported to be satisfactory[4].

(2)   Linearity: The measuring range must be defined clearly as must the range of values covered by the test (normal range, borderline, pathological range, extreme values, decision limits, alarm limits). It is desirable to have clear instructions for the actions to be taken if the result is out of linearity (dilution, prolongation of reaction time etc.)[5,6].

(3)   Imprecision: Current goals for imprecision are based upon biological variation. The analytical goal is that the standard deviation of clinical biochemistry tests should be less than or equal to one half of the average intra-individual biological variation. The imprecision should be indicated in the same units as the quantity assessed (result) rather than in CV percentage.

(4)   Inaccuracy: Methods used in clinical biochemistry laboratories should have no bias whatsoever[4]. This statement is valid for decentralized laboratories too. The test results

from different laboratories must be directly comparable.

(5)   Quality control: Since no procedure is perfectly stable, a means must be supplied, as part of the method, to control chemical and instrumental instability. Monitoring variances and correcting the sources of deviation, including error detection, diagnosis and remedial action form part of operator instruction.

REAGENTS

For some time, 'dry reagents' have been available for urine testing (single- and multi-sticks). Recently dip-sticks and slides for serum and blood testing have considerably increased the test programme. Together with prepacked reagents for closed systems, an almost complete clinical chemistry test programme is covered. For all these reagents, the same or stronger regulations as for wet-chemistry must be applied.

Labelling

As diagnostic reagents become subject to performance standards, these products have to be manufactured according to the criteria of good manufacturing practices (GMP). The ECCLS Standard for the Labelling of Clinical Laboratory Materials must be followed[7]. Package inserts, product information and user instructions must be written in the language commonly used in centralized and decentralized laboratories.

Storage conditions and maintenance

Although the production of reagents, equipment and other materials needed for the performance of laboratory tasks has increasingly involved production capabilities external to the laboratory itself, the laboratory must still assume responsibility for the quality and integrity of the materials and equipment it employs.

Even with no noticeable deterioration of the reagent site, reagents must not be used after their expiration date. Reagents should be stored in their original containers and protected from light and humidity[8].

ORGANIZATION AND STANDARDIZATION

For practical and economical reasons, decentralized testing in a hospital should be organized by the central laboratory manager. The staff performing the decentralized clinical laboratory testing may follow the continuous education programme of the central laboratory staff, at least for the subjects the decentralized laboratory is involved in.

The use of simplified methods may not cause problems in standardization if, as is the case in urine testing, the method is also widely used in centralized laboratories such that other methods become obsolete. This is unfortunately not the case with many tests performed in serum. For example the reaction conditions in 'dry chemistry' cannot follow the IFCC recommendations for enzyme determinations.

It must be stated that the results produced by recommended standard methods and results produced by simplified techniques are directly comparable.

REFERENCES

1. Boutwell JH and Mater A, (1973). Diagnostic Methods. Proceedings: International Conference on Standardization of Diagnostic Materials, pp 27-41.
2. Broughton PMG et al, (1985). Guidelines for Kit Evaluation. 2nd Draft. ECCLS Document Vol 5, No 1.
3. Horder M and Jorgensen PJ, (1982). Die Bedeutung der Lyse für den Nachweis Zellulärer Urinbestandteile. Das 'Teststreifensieb', Boehringer Mannheim, 37-44.
4. Fraser CG, (1983). The Future Small Lab. IFCC NEWS No 35, p.4.
5. Richterich R, Greiner R and Küffer H, (1973). Analysatoren in der Klinischen Chemie. III. Beurteilungs-Kriterien und Fehlerquellen. Z Klin Chem Klin Biochem, 11, 65-75.
6. von Klein-Wiesenberg A, von Boroviczény K-G and Merten R, (1977). Medizin und Einheitengesetz. INSTAND, Triltsch: Düsseldorf.
7. Storring PL et al, (1985). Standard for the Labelling of Clinical Laboratory Materials. ECCLS Document Vol 2, No 3.
8. Free HM et al, (1986). Dry Reagent Strip Tests. NCCLS Draft Guidelines.

Discussion

Mill   Dr Küffer used the term clinical usefulness but Dr Browning says methods giving unsatisfactory results cannot be tolerated. Rapid tests may have a Coefficient of Variation of 10-20% but may save life. We in industry cannot get the answer when we ask for figures on clinical relevance. In our experience clinicians just don't know.

Dybkaer   The whole question hinges on the clinical

situation which varies from case to case and it is impossible to provide a generalized answer.

Mitchell   Years ago the IFCC expert panel on instrumentation tried to provide an answer for industry on this. A typical reply to a query was obtained in India from a famous surgeon who said his most urgent requirement was to obtain an instrument which told him whether the haemoglobin level in blood was above or below 4 g/100 ml.

Haeckel   The question of speed is sometimes exaggerated. An investigation recently conducted of the time taken by the ward to act on a result showed that such time was at least 50% of the time taken to obtain the result.

Hjelm   Much more effort is needed to improve instruments themselves for decentralization and to solve the problem of expired reagents.

Dybkaer   Work of this kind is already being carried out. There is a new glucometer which recalibrates according to the batch number of strips being used. I feel sure that other clever systems will be devised in the near future.

Gilhuus-Moe   I see two types of home testing. The first is the pregnancy-type test which is a one-off used on one occasion only by the patient. The second type includes the tests used by diabetics where a life-long commitment is involved. Here the patient is very keen to become involved and is interested in the results because they are life saving.

Dybkaer   Our patient this morning was highly intelligent and motivated but we must cope with many others who are not.

Gilhuus-Moe   Even she only applies quality control once a year.

Leighton   All present systems depend on colour change and this is very difficult to control. Controls are difficult or impossible to obtain for example for Strep. cultures for bacteriology. Some kits are produced by unscrupulous manufacturers and we must have some sort of a Kite Mark possibly operated by ECCLS to guarantee quality.

Dybkaer   We should look to a system where no instrument can go to a GP unless it has been passed by some organization. FDA do something like this. Also there should be a good connection with a central testing facility.

Leighton We are associated in our laboratory with some 400 GPs. How can we see them all?

Dybkaer In Odense they have approximately 100 GPs but work a control system for the instruments which the GPs use.

10

Safety of Personnel and Environment

Roger D Jennings

INTRODUCTION

Safety is of major importance in any laboratory and laboratory procedure, but where such procedures are undertaken outside a major laboratory, especially in an area not purpose-designed for such work or by staff not specifically trained in laboratory techniques, safety becomes even more important.

This paper considers some of the requirements for the safe performance of laboratory testing in decentralized areas and the possible hazards which may arise. Many considerations apply equally well to testing in a central laboratory as to tests performed outside, but even so they are worth repeating in this context.

One very important contribution to the safety of the decentralized test area is for one person to be officially designated as having responsibility for all operations in that area. Unsupervised use will always lead to problems.

SPECIFIC REQUIREMENTS FOR SAFETY

Test repertoire

The first point to consider is the limiting of the repertoire of tests to be performed. Table 10.1 suggests a list of the types of test which might be performed depending on the particular location where testing takes place. The situation is changing rapidly and analytical techniques for many other assays are being developed, or will soon be developed, enabling these to be undertaken safely in a decentralized laboratory area or even at home. At present however it would be most unwise, for example, to attempt the measurement of a trace metal in a doctor's office since this would require the use of a flammable gas, or the measurement of a hormone by a technique using radioisotopes in a similar situation.

Table 10.1 Repertoire of tests which may be carried out in decentralized testing areas

Test area	Test types
Satellite laboratory staffed by laboratory personnel	Most chemical pathology and haematology tests Microbiology procedures except those requiring a Class 1 safety cabinet
Ward side room laboratory or doctor's office staffed by non-laboratory personnel	Chemical pathology and haematology tests not involving hazardous reagents e.g. ISE Na/K, 'dry chemistry' procedures, blood gases, bilirubinometer, haemoglobinometer, occult blood Limited serology
Home monitoring by patients	'Stick' tests Pregnancy tests

Training

Once an appropriate repertoire of tests is identified all staff who will be involved in these tests must receive comprehensive, formal training. This does not mean passing instructions from one operator to another by word of mouth. What is required is a documented training programme which demonstrates that the trainee understands what he or she has been taught and that he or she is competent to perform the operations required. The operator must satisfactorily complete a formal assessment of competence before undertaking analysis on patients' samples. The results of this assessment must be recorded. Steps should be taken to ensure that only trained operators are allowed to perform tests or other procedures.

Documentation

One very important contribution to safety is the clear, concise and adequate documentation of all procedures. It is also essential that such documentation be updated as soon as any procedure is altered. Staff should not be permitted to alter any procedure unless that alteration has been approved and documented by the test area supervisor or his designated deputy.

POTENTIAL HAZARDS

Microbiological safety

There are several problems to consider concerning microbiological safety. Any human sample is potentially infectious and must be handled carefully but this does not imply that everything must be handled in a Class 1 safety cabinet! The risk of acquiring AIDS, in the laboratory is for example. very small indeed, but of course it would not be appropriate to handle specimens from a patient with viral haemorrhagic fever without special precautions, in either a central laboratory or a specially designed mobile isolator.

Elementary hygiene is, of course, essential. Eating, drinking, smoking, applying cosmetics and mouth pipetting in the laboratory area must all be prohibited. Suitable protective clothing should be worn at all times in the laboratory area but it should not be worn outside. To minimize the amount of manipulation required, analytical procedures should use whole blood. Where it is essential to use plasma or serum, mechanical or chemical aids to separation should be employed. If shaking, mixing or centrifuging of the sample or reaction tube is required then the tube must be capped. Spillages must be mopped up immediately and the area involved decontaminated. All waste must be disposed of safely. Infectious waste should be autoclaved or incinerated. All 'sharps' should be disposed of in a special container.

Chemical hazards

Chemical hazards should not be a great problem if the technical procedures which are to be used are chosen carefully. As mentioned before, no procedure should use flammable gases or radioisotopes. In addition they should not involve the use of corrosive, toxic, carcinogenic or flammable chemicals.

Electrical and mechanical hazards

These can be minimized. Firstly by the proper selection of equipment and secondly by adequate maintenance. No equipment should be purchased unless it complies with a national or international safety standard. Before it is introduced into the test area it should undergo an inspection by a competent engineer. It should then be introduced into a maintenance programme. This might be merely a brief, periodic inspection but might involve a full maintenance check by the equipment manufacturer or his agent. Staff should not be permitted to interfere with any equipment but be told to report any faults as soon as they occur, for rectification by suitably trained personnel.

CONCLUSIONS

Clearly all that is required is to put good laboratory practice into operation. However, when staff involved in testing are trained in other disciplines or, indeed, when the patient carrying out tests on himself is untrained, then additional care is required to ensure that the safety implications of all procedures are fully understood by those who are to carry them out.

Discussion

Dybkaer	Mr Jennings pointed out that a lot of training is necessary. Where should this be done, who should do it and what should be the syllabus?
Jennings	Many manufacturers are willing to provide training and central laboratories also have a role. We should consider what training is involved and include other aspects than just safety.
Dybkaer	It would also be desirable to carry out periodic retraining but manufacturers would not be able to do this.
Martin	But they should be able to provide training material to the hospital authorities.
Fagraeus	What about infectious samples? Many countries have rules for central laboratories which could be applied.
Jennings	This hazard may be less than in the main laboratory since the person carrying out the test is more likely to be aware of the patient's problems.
Elliott	All equipment should be decontaminated before it is returned to industry for any reason at all.
Wilde	Yes, but it is the responsibility of the manufacturer to state exactly how this should be done.
Jennings	In ten years time all equipment which we use for these purposes could be 'dry' but until then we should lay down procedures and

Elliott

manufacturers should help.
Manufacturers should know what materials can and cannot be used in this sort of equipment but the onus for safety from contamination should finally rest with the health authority involved.

11

Patient Reception, Preparation, Specimen Handling and Data Flow

Colin E Wilde

INTRODUCTION

There are many reasons why clinicians require test results on the body fluids of their patients. They may be to confirm a tentative diagnosis, to help solve differential diagnostic problems, to monitor therapy, to assess prognosis, to screen for latent disease, or to use for an epidemiological programme, for research or for teaching. Decentralized testing may be used for any of these. If a test result is to be of value it must be free from error and ambiguity. If it is likely to be affected by any factors or conditions to which the patient or specimen has been subjected before analysis these factors must be taken into careful consideration before a result is accepted and in the interpretation of the results.

With centralized testing there is usually a complex chain of events following the initiation of a request by a clinician before a medically useful result is provided. This chain can involve many different processes and many different people including clinician, patient, nurses, porters, drivers, reception staff, technical staff, scientific staff, clerks and secretaries. There are many pre- and post-analytical factors which arise during this chain of events and one of the attractions of decentralized testing, which is of course closer to the patient, is the removal of some of these steps which may influence the result. Thus decentralized testing should more easily enable the correct identification of patient and specimen throughout the process, the reduction of the time interval between specimen collection and analysis, the removal of adverse environmental conditions to which the specimen is subjected during the period between specimen collection and analysis, and the rapid timely transmission of the correct result to the right source.

Decentralized testing does not remove all the pre- and post-analytical factors which affect test results and it has the disadvantage of the involvement of a much greater number of testing sites and many more personnel performing the testing. These personnel are unlikely to have the necessary basic training for a proper awareness of the factors which might affect the results of tests and which ought to be taken into account in the interpretation of the results. This paper outlines some of these factors at the patient reception stage, during patient preparation, during specimen handling and in data transmission and recording.

PATIENT RECEPTION

Facilities must be provided in the patient reception area to enable the correct type of specimen to be easily and conveniently collected with minimum inconvenience to the doctor or nurse and minimum stress to the patient. Short-term stress can affect the levels of many important diagnostic constituents in body fluids and it is important that the surroundings are pleasant and that the patient is relaxed and at ease prior to and during specimen collection.

The reception area must have adequate washing facilities so that if necessary the patient may wash prior to specimen collection to avoid contamination with commensal organisms in urine or possibly in wound discharges or skin biopsies. The washing facilities are also needed to enable the person collecting the specimen to remove immediately any contamination with potentially infectious body fluids or exudates, or with material which may contaminate the specimen. Toilet facilities are necessary for the collection of urine and faecal specimens by patients and for their general convenience.

A bed or couch must be available as certain investigations require the patient to be recumbent. The posture of the patient may affect the circulating levels of the constituent being investigated or may be important for the convenient collection of the specimen. There should also be facilities for the patient to lie down if needing to recover or feeling unwell.

A phlebotomy chair with adjustable arm rests must be provided for patients' comfort and for easy access to the patient by the phlebotomist.

The patient reception area should be equipped with the necessary technical equipment for collection of specimens. This will include sterile swabs, syringes, needles and a range of specimen containers with appropriate preservatives or anticoagulants. It will also include antiseptic swabs for cleaning venepuncture sites, quick release tourniquets and a sphygmomanometer. In the event of a possible infection risk e.g. from a hepatitis B or HIV positive patient, gloves, eye visors and impermeable aprons or gowns should be available for the operator. There must be suitable containers for the disposal of used needles, syringes and swabs, and disinfectants should be available in case of spillage.

There must also be facilities to interview the patient and to record positive patient identification together with other details such as age, sex, drug therapy, time of day and type of specimen which are relevant to the interpretation of the test result.

PATIENT PREPARATION

Stress

The results of tests, particularly those on circulating blocd constituents, may be altered if the patient is anxious or tense. Ideally the patient should be made to feel relaxed and at ease before any specimen is collected. This is equally true for an ambulant outpatient or for a patient admitted to a critical care area, where rapid tests might be most usefully performed, but where the patient is likely to be under considerable stress. Some tests which are significantly affected by the stress factor are blood glucose, growth hormone, prolactin, cortisol, catecholamines, coagulation factors and blood count.

Dietary factors

The dietary state of the patient may also be relevant to the test being performed. Significant changes in the concentration of blood constituents may occur after meals, particularly that of glucose and triglycerides but also that of urea, phosphate, iron, uric acid and alkaline phosphatase. Some tests require the patient to have fasted overnight, e.g. glucose tolerance tests or plasma lipids, if meaningful results are to be obtained. If the patient has undergone prolonged fasting, clotting factors, some enzymes, bilirubin, proteins and glucose levels will be altered.

Alcohol and smoking

Alcohol consumption and smoking may also produce misleading results for some tests. Alcohol effects are complex depending on whether intake is habitual or whether it has been taken after a meal, but a 50% increase in blood glucose can be recorded after alcohol ingestion and changes in uric acid, gamma glutamyl transferase, lactate and amylase are likely. Smoking affects lipase, amylase, cholesterol and glucose and also gastric absorption as in a glucose tolerance test.

Drug therapy

Drug therapy is the most frequent cause of misinterpretation of test results. Some drugs interfere with the analytical methodology but a greater number of problems are caused by physiological changes which alter the test result and for some investigations drug therapy must be discontinued prior to the test. Such drug interactions are very numerous and well-documented. For instance, at least 80 drugs may cause in vitro or in vivo plasma glucose test interactions and over 50 have been shown to alter the results of urine glucose assays. The obvious effect of antibiotic treatment on microbiological tests is another which often gives misleading negative results if treatment is started before testing and the time is not carefully recorded. Drug interference may be specific for a particular methodology whereas another method for the same test may not be so affected. A knowledge of the principle of the test is therefore necessary in addition to a general awareness of the possibility of drug interference.

Posture

The position of the patient before and during specimen collection is important when measuring certain blood constituents. There are considerable changes in levels, mainly due to haemoconcentration or haemodilution, depending on whether the patient has been standing, sitting or lying down prior to specimen collection. Such changes mainly affect haemoglobin, proteins, albumin, enzymes and lipids. Ideally, for any blood test the patient should be supine or sitting for at least 15 minutes prior to blood collection.

Circadian rhythms

Many body fluid constituent levels follow circadian rhythms and therefore it is wise to take specimens at standard times during the day, preferably early in the morning between 0700 h and 0900 h. Significant rhythms are shown by iron, cortisol, acid phosphatase, glucose tolerance and urinary sodium and potassium. Another area where timing of specimen collection is important is in therapeutic drug monitoring where the time interval between drug dosage and analysis of circulating levels is critical to the interpretation of the result.

Exercise

Exhausting muscular work up to 3 days before sampling alters the levels of creatine kinase, LDH, potassium, glucose, lactate, creatinine and clotting factors and rather more gentle exercise, including excessive flexing of the forearm before venepuncture, causes changes in potassium, lactate, glucose, proteins and some enzymes. In the case of venepuncture any forearm exercise should be avoided.

DEALINGS WITH PATIENTS, SPECIMENS AND DATA

Medical procedures

Medical procedures such as massage, palpation and even injections can cause local changes in blood constituents so that creatine kinase may rise with any of these and acid phosphatase may be misleadingly high after palpation in the prostatic area. Another frequent cause of erroneous blood levels of many components is specimen-taking from a catheterized arm being infused with intravenous fluids.

Nature of the specimen

The site of specimen collection and the type of specimen needed will depend on the question which is being asked, the analyte to be measured, the amount of sample needed, and the anatomical situation. If the lower respiratory tract is being investigated and sputum is required, the results will be misleading if the specimen is mainly saliva. Female gonorrhoea is best investigated in samples from the cervix or urethral discharge rather than the vagina, as gonococci do not thrive in the acidic conditions. Early morning urine specimens are likely to be more concentrated and therefore better for detecting some constituents. On the other hand, this concentration effect may be misleading and a quantitative measurement on a timed urine specimen may give more useful information provided that it is carefully collected and the volume recorded accurately. A clean mid-stream urine specimen is essential for most microbiological work and the patient should wash carefully prior to collection to minimize contamination with commensal organisms.

For blood specimens there is a choice of arterial, venous or capillary blood. Venous blood is influenced by the metabolism and haemodynamics of the region it drains and capillary blood will to an even greater extent vary depending on the capillary bed from which it is derived. Venous blood is generally sampled from the forearm and capillary blood from the outer plantar surface of the foot or the heel region in young children or the lower ear or the fingertip in adults. There will be concentration differences between these specimens particularly for metabolites such as glucose and lactate. It is particularly important that specimens taken as a series in one patient are collected in identical fashion.

Whether the sampling is venous or capillary the site should be cleaned thoroughly by swabbing with 70% isopropyl alcohol or a similar preparation. The site should be allowed to dry because of the danger of haemolysis and patient discomfort. The composition of capillary specimens is influenced by the temperature of the skin, by the depth of incision, by dilution with tissue fluids and by partial coagulation of the blood during collection. The use of the tourniquet during venepuncture to enhance distension of the veins is normal practice but prolonged application causes haemoconcentration with pronounced increases in the levels of proteins, enzymes, albumin, potassium, calcium, lipids, haemoglobin and packed cell volume. Training programmes should ensure an awareness of these problems and as a general rule a tourniquet not exceeding systolic blood pressure should be applied not longer than 1 minute prior to venepuncture.

Special precautions should be taken according to local safety codes when collecting specimens from patients perceived to be an infection risk.

SPECIMEN HANDLING

Many of the problems of specimen handling, in terms of staff safety or sample deterioration over lengthy time periods at inappropriate temperatures during storage, transport or transfer to the laboratory, might be expected to be circumvented by performing tests closer to the patient. However, operators should be fully aware of the potential sources of error and danger to their own person caused by poor specimen handling technique even over short periods of time. As it is often a wise precaution to preserve some specimen in the event of further investigations being required, careful handling and preservation of the specimen is essential.

Delay before analysis

The time interval between specimen collection and testing should be as short as possible. In the analysis of blood gases, PO_2 changes significantly when left for 20 min even at 4°C, and 7% of glucose in blood without preservative disappears during the first hour. Longer delays enable red cell constituents to leak out of the cells, affecting the levels or analysis of a number of plasma constituents, most notably potassium. Evaporation in small volumes of body fluids, or from swabs for microbiological testing, may produce significantly altered values or loss of bacterial viability if drying out occurs. Indeed, if delay is likely before testing, bacteriological swabs should be immersed in an appropriate transport medium and addition of preservatives may be necessary, for example to inhibit red cell glycolytic enzymes prior to glucose assay or in 24 hour urine specimens to inhibit bacterial growth. All containers must be well stoppered and stored at the appropriate temperature. Urine specimens for microbiological investigations should be dealt with immediately as urine is a good bacteriological culture medium and multiplication of the organisms, or overgrowth of contaminating bacteria, may produce misleading results or spoil the investigation.

DEALINGS WITH PATIENTS, SPECIMENS AND DATA

Contamination

Contamination of the specimen should be carefully avoided. No antiseptics or other antimicrobial agents should come into contact with specimens for microbiological investigations and all specimen containers for such tests should be sterile before use. Many tests are now performed with very small volumes of sample, perhaps 10 μL, and are very sensitive. It is relatively easy for significant contamination to occur from the fingers. As little as 1 μL of a 20% glucose infusion solution contaminating a small capillary collection tube can falsely elevate a blood glucose reading by 10 mmol/L and similar amounts of disinfectant or antiseptic may interfere with many biochemical tests. The sample used for testing must always be fully representative of the specimen and this is normally achieved by careful mixing before an aliquot is taken for testing. Exposure of specimens to light should be avoided particularly if bilirubin is to be measured.

Haemolysis

Haemolysis in blood specimens may occur in a number of ways, such as by poor specimen collection, by expelling blood from the syringe too quickly, by contamination with antiseptic agents, by vigorous mixing, by centrifuging too quickly or at too high a temperature, or by leaving the blood too long before analysis or removal of cells. This leads to the presence of red cell constituents in the plasma or serum and causes increases in levels of potassium, phosphate, haemoglobin and interference with some enzyme assays. Considerable errors can occur when a bilirubinometer is used to analyse haemolysed specimens. Results from haemolysed blood specimens should always be interpreted with care.

Anticoagulants

Many tests designed for use in wards or clinics accept whole blood but others require plasma or serum. The use of an anticoagulant to produce plasma has advantages in that the cells may be separated without delay and there is less likelihood of haemolysis. However, the type and amount of anticoagulant must be chosen with care. Thus blood collected into tri potassium EDTA tubes, commonly used for haematological investigation, will not be suitable for potassium or calcium determinations. The addition of excessive amounts of heparin to arterial blood samples can produce significant errors in the results of pH, pCO_2 and pO_2 measurements and too much EDTA will produce artefactual changes in red cell morphology. It is very important that the correct amount of blood is always placed in containers containing anticoagulant and that gentle mixing takes place to ensure solution without excessive shaking which will lead to cell lysis.

Centrifugation

If plasma or serum is required, removal of cells by centrifugation may be necessary. This should be performed to clearly defined instructions at a standard speed and time without undue acceleration or deceleration to minimize haemolytic effects. A serum separator may be helpful to ease separation and prevent remixing.

Safety

In the handling of specimens the safety of the operator and other personnel and patients must always be borne in mind even when the patient or specimen is not expected to present an infection risk. Care must be taken not to contaminate the sides of containers or any part of the environment with specimen, and if any is spilt it must be cleaned up immediately with suitable disinfectant. If a particular infection risk is perceived special precautions for specimen handling must be observed.

Sample identification

If the specimen is transferred to any type of container prior to the test, the container must be labelled clearly with the patient identification and if possible the type of specimen, time etc.

DATA HANDLING

Patient demographics

Full patient identification including the patient's family name, given names, address, personal health number, date of birth and source of request should be recorded unless the test is to be performed immediately and the result entered directly into the patient's record. If the result is entered into an electronic data handling system great care must be exercised to ensure that it is entered into the correct patient's records and under the correct test heading.

Drug therapy and other relevant information

Details of all current drug therapy should be noted as should the time of day. Where relevant the posture of the patient before and during specimen collection and details of dietary state and other special circumstances such as smoking or ethanol intake should be noted.

Calculating results

Any calculations which may have to be performed, including the use of dilution factors, must be recorded at the time of analysis. If the equipment produces a hardcopy printout this should be attached to the report form to minimize transcription errors.

Reporting data

The units of measurement and the method of analysis must accompany the result as either may vary in different parts of the hospital or other localities. Errors in interpretation due to bias between different methods is one of the greatest dangers of decentralized testing and it is essential to report carefully the exact nature of the test result, its quantity and the units in which that quantity is expressed.

All results are compared with reference points or reference ranges and these vary with age, sex, time of day and many of the preanalytical factors which have been discussed. Provision must be made either by written tables or with the help of computers to enable interpretation of the result against the correct reference range, taking into account any known interfering factors.

A list of test results must be kept in the laboratory and must be easily available should the result not have reached the source of request and in case of any query. Arrangements must be made to have unexpected abnormal results checked by the central laboratory or to arrange for further follow-up tests to be performed to confirm the findings.

CONCLUSIONS

This presentation has attempted to cover the main criteria which must be considered during patient reception, preparation, specimen handling and data flow for decentralized testing. It has been concerned mainly with factors which introduce errors affecting the results and interpretation of tests. It has not attempted to define those factors which are likely to be clinically relevant in particular circumstances as these circumstances will vary widely. The purpose for which tests are performed will differ and the availability of other clinical information will also vary.

Although the extent of the influence of these factors on test results will not always be clinically relevant, it is important that standards for their control be set and followed wherever possible and that clinicians and medical auxillaries performing decentralized testing be fully aware of the factors affecting the tests they perform. It is to fill this need that ECCLS guidelines are currently being prepared.

Discussion

Elliott	In the preparation of ECCLS standards by Dr Dybkaer's subcommittees, should they define all known relevant factors or just draw attention to them?
Wilde	It is impossible to list every known factor but it is useful to produce guidelines giving important examples so that those in charge of decentralized areas can be aware of this type of effect and look at the factors most important to their work.
Martin	Are there any other standards in this area already?
Wilde	There is much in the literature but it is not coordinated in such a way as to be accessible to those involved in decentralized testing.

12

Quality Assurance, Teaching and Training

Dolphe Kutter

INTRODUCTION

Quality control is an absolute necessity in clinical chemistry regardless of where, by whom and by what methods it is performed. This certainly applies to decentralized testing in the hospital.

Today specialized industries offer a wide variety of simplified diagnostics meant for analysts who have not been professionally trained. There is no reason why these technical facilities should not be used in the hospital wards. The main clinical situations which call for decentralized testing are summarized in Table 12.1. There is no need to transfer to the ward other parameters such as cholesterol, triglycerides, and even other 'emergency' parameters such as CK, AST and ALT. Some diagnostic systems currently available for decentralized use are presented in Table 12.2. This paper does not consider the problem of blood gas analysers but is restricted to truly simplified systems.

The problem of quality assurance of rapid and simplified diagnostics should be considered from two points of view. Firstly, the user needs to know about the clinical performance of the test and whether it is able to give the precise clinical information that is required. This question can only be answered after thorough clinical trials. Secondly, it is necessary to know the analytical performance of the test and whether it performs according to the specifications stated by the manufacturers. It is this aspect of performance which will be specifically considered in this paper.

IMPORTANT CHARACTERISTICS OF TEST SYSTEMS

Qualitative tests

For the qualitative tests, among which are most of the urine test strips, the most important characteristics are their sensitivity and their specificity. Owing to the highly variable chemical composition

Table 12.1 Clinical situations in which decentralized testing may be useful

Situation	Analysis	Analyst
I. Emergencies:		
Comatous states	Blood glucose	
	Blood urea and NH_3	
Severe abdominal pain	Amylase in urine	Physician
	Lipase in plasma	Nursing staff
Respiratory distress	Blood gases	
II. Monitoring		
Therapy and follow-up	Blood glucose	Nursing staff
of diabetes	Glycosuria	Patient
Intensive care	Plasma Na + K + NH_3	
	Urine specific gravity	
	Blood gases	Nursing staff
Renal unit	Blood urea	
	Plasma K	
III. Relief of the work-load of the central laboratory	Urinary screening	Nursing staff

of urine, it is impossible to characterize sensitivity by just one value. It must be seen from a statistical point of view. When plotting the percentage of positive reactions against metabolite concentration a typical sensitivity curve is obtained, which should be constant for a well-standardized reagent (Figure 12.1). Such a curve is characterized by two essential points: maximum sensitivity (S_{10}) represents the concentration detectable in 10% of a large number of specimens. These are the specimens with the most favourable reaction conditions. Practical sensitivity (S_{90}) is the concentration detectable under more usual conditions in 90% of a large number of specimens. The slope of the curve, given by the difference between S_{10} and S_{90} depends upon the influence of urinary constituents upon the reaction. Maximum efficiency is obtained when the sensitivity curve comes as close as possible to the area representing the normal population without S_{10} dropping into it. In Figure 12.1 completely normal people are represented by a Gaussian curve. This figure also shows that a certain number of false negatives may be unavoidable depending on the slope and the position of the curve.

Important information concerning the specificity of a test can be deduced from the reaction mechanism, which should always be disclosed. It makes it possible to foresee a certain number of interferences, whose importance must be determined in model experiments. Other interferences are detected during the clinical trial and later on in clinical practice. The list of possible non-specific reactions should be regularly updated by the producers and be communicated to the users.

Table 12.2 Diagnostic systems available for use in the hospital ward

Type of test	Analysis time	Type of evaluation
Qualitative single and multiple test strips for urinalysis	1-2 min	Visual Reflectometry (Urotron[R], Clinitek[R], Rapimat[R], Aution[R])

Quantitative test strips for whole blood analysis	3 min	Visual (Haemoglukotest 20-800[R], Glucostix, Visidex[R], Azostix[R])
		Reflectometry:
		  One parameter reflectometer (Glucometer[R], Reflocheck[R], Glucosot[R] etc.)
		  Multiparameter relectometer (Reflotron[R], Vision[R], Hemascope[R] etc.)

	15 min	Specific reflectometer (blood ammonia checker: Dai-ichi Kyoto)
Blood gas meters, whole blood electrolyte analysers	5 min	Specific electrodes
Quantitative test strips for determinations on plasma or serum	15 min	Multiparameter reflectometer (seralyser[R])

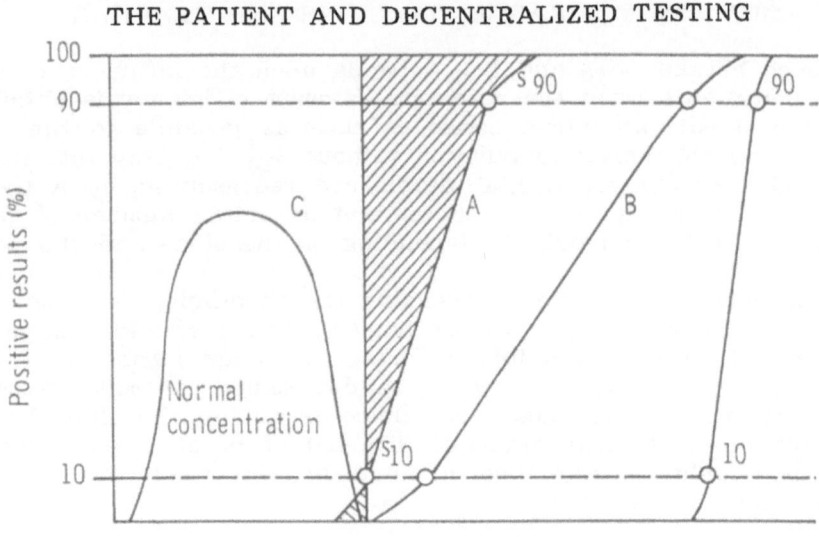

Figure 12.1 Types of sensitivity curves.

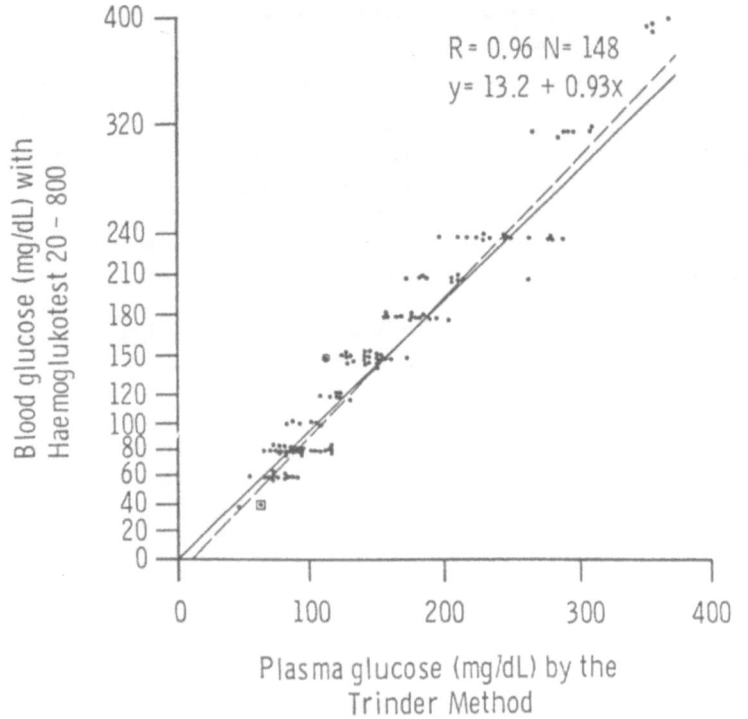

Figure 12.2 Results of Haemoglukotest 20-800[R](Boehringer-Mannheim) showing good correlation with the reference method and absence of systematic error.

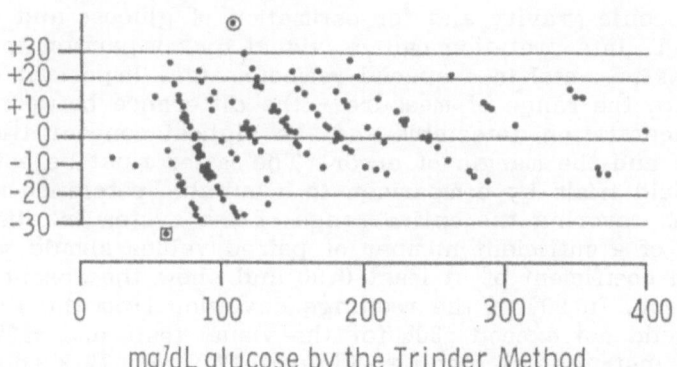

Figure 12.3 Percentage deviation of Haemoglukotest 20-800[R] from reference method.

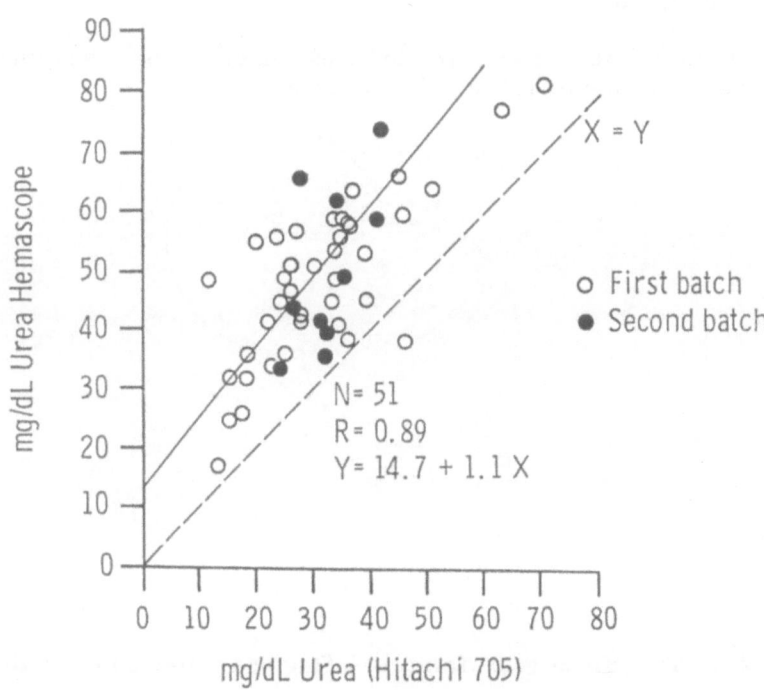

Figure 12.4 Determination of urea by Hemascope in comparison to the reference determination on the Hitachi 705.

Quantitative tests

Quantitative test strips have been designed for determination of
urinary specific gravity and for estimation of glucose and urea in
whole blood. Interpretation can be visual by comparison to a colour
scale or instrumental in a special reflectometer. Important characteristics are the range of measure - the difference between the
lowest concentration detectable and the highest concentration dis-
cernable - and the margin of error. The latter must be established
in large field trials by comparison to a suitable reference method,
with values covering the entire range of the system. Statistical
evaluation of a sufficient number of paired values should yield a
correlation coefficient of at least 0.90 and show the absence of systematic error. In 90% of the readings deviation from the reference
values should not exceed ±30% for the visual tests and ±15% for
tests with instrumental reading. Figures 12.2 and 12.3 show an acceptable status of the visual glucose test strip Haemoglukotest 20-
800 (Boehringer, Mannheim). For the blood urea test strip read in
Hemascope[R] (Dai-Chi-Kyoto) heavy systematic overestimation is
evident (Figure 12.4).

QUALITY ASSURANCE

Internal quality assurance procedures should be designed to
monitor the areas identified in Figure 12.5.

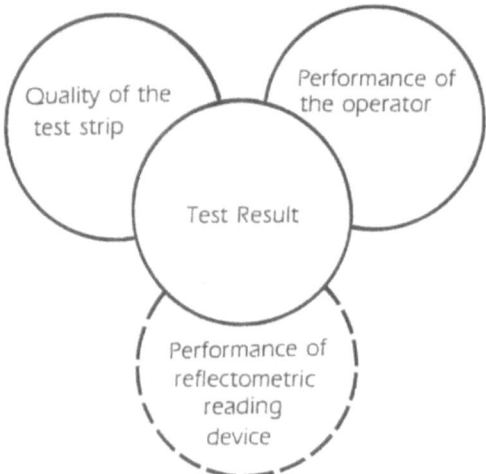

Figure 12.5 The three main factors influencing the test result.

The first question concerns the operator: does he execute
the test according to the instructions and - when reading the test

by eye - does he have acceptable colour vision? It must be remembered that decentralized testing often involves inexperienced operators. It is astonishing to see how even the simplest instructions are followed incorrectly. Good colour vision may not be taken for granted. We have been able to demonstrate by means of a very simple, home-made system that many people lack the ability to distinguish between subtle differences of colour without being colour-blind.

The second question concerns the test material itself: does it perform according to the characteristic target values established in the clinical trial? Defects may occur during production and remain unnoticed despite the producer's internal control system. Possible deterioration may be caused by poor transport and storage conditions. The shelf-life of such products is another problem. The unopened package must be guaranteed by an expiry date. This does not, however, apply to the package once opened. In this case deterioration may occur especially if the package has remained open over a longer period of time.

A third question concerns the reflectometric reading device. Improper function - often caused by faults in maintenance or low power supply - and incorrect calibration must be excluded.

Control materials

It is essential that control materials imitate natural conditions as much as possible. This is not generally the case for synthetic control specimens. Artificial 'grey strips' may be used for checking the performance of a reflectometric reading device. They offer of course no guarantee that the test strips will function adequately.

(a) Urine: The commercial availability of control urines in stabilized liquid form, tablets, lyophilates, strips and capsules is limited, and the products are usually restricted to a few metabolites. Metabolite concentrations are often high and detectable even by poorly performing reagents, and may be present in unnatural forms such as free bilirubin instead of conjugated bilirubin. Others are replaced by artificial substitutes.

Urine tests performed in the hospital ward may be controlled by the central laboratory in two ways: adequate urine pools may be prepared by the central laboratory and distributed to the wards. We are using two pools which are kept deep-frozen in 5 mL portions. For the first pool we have diluted a urine specimen extremely rich in urobilinogen with 'Atkins'-urine containing ketones to a final concentration of 2 mg/dL urobilinogen. This specimen is spiked with 20 mg/dL human albumin and stabilized with 100 mg/dL ascorbic acid. Even in the frozen state urobilinogen is not stable without this additive. The second pool is an icteric specimen diluted to 0.5 mg/dL with normal urine and spiked with 50 mg/dL glucose, 20 erythrocytes/μL and 20 leukocytes/μL. Erythrocytes are added as haemolyzed blood, leukocytes from a urine specimen containing a high concentration of leukocytes.

Table 12.3 Test strip quality control using the median values obtained by the reference method for the different concentration ranges.

Test results:	trace – +	++	+++
Leukocytes per µL by	0	0	218
chamber counting:	0	0	582
	0	0	832 832
	0	8	840
	0	11	2538
	0	27	
	0	35	
	0	37	
	0	40	
	0	43	
	0	43 43	
	0	43	
	0	43	
	0	48	
	5	59	
	11	59	
	16 16	75	
	21	96	
	21	123	
	21	150	
	21	165	
	21		
	21		
	27		
	37		
	37		
	43		
	43		
	67		
	96		
	176		
	779		

If a positive reaction obtained at the wards leads to quantitative follow-up, the results may be used for quality control. Leukocyte test strips provide a good example. When applying the 'test strip sieve', every positive reaction for protein, blood or leukocyte esterase is followed by quantitative chamber counting. Statistical comparison of the leukocytes counts corresponding to 'trace - +' reaction on the strip should yield values of the same order of magnitude as was determined in the clinical field trial for this test strip. Table 12.3 shows results for the leukocyte test area of Combur-9-Test[R] (Boehringer Mannheim). The median value of 16 leukocytes/μL was also found in the clinical trial indicating that this test must be in order. When reading the same test in the Urotron RL9 the median value for the '+' results was 107 leukocytes/μL, indicating gross underestimation.

(b) Plasma or serum: Quality control is easier for systems determining plasma or serum metabolites. Commercial test sera or lyophilates may be supplied by the central laboratory. Their viscosity must however be similar to that of serum or plasma. Specific target values should be available.

(c) Whole blood: Whole blood methods cannot be controlled with test sera or plasma. Test strips are designed to restrict the reaction to plasma by excluding the red cells from the reactive surface by semipermeable membranes of suitable porosity. However experience shows that the red cells slow down the penetration of plasma into the reactive area (Figure 12.6). This is why results

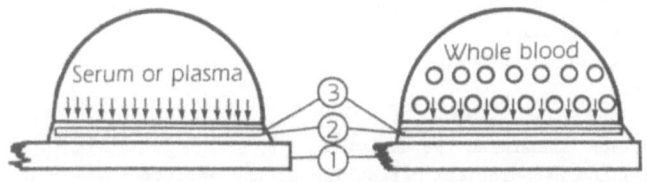

Figure 12.6 Penetration of glucose into the test area when using plasma or serum (A) and whole blood (B).
1 = plastic strip. 2 = reactive area. 3 = semipermeable membrane.

obtained with the whole blood are always lower and not comparable to determination in plasma. This problem is almost impossible to solve in office practice. Solution is easy in the hospital. An aliquot of blood drawn at the ward can be mixed with a suitable anticoagulant and sent directly to the central laboratory for control by the reference method. Results obtained at the ward must lie within a certain limit of tolerance.

TEACHING AND TRAINING

Acceptable results in the ward can only be obtained after thorough teaching and training. The teaching programme should cover the topics listed in Table 12.4. Theory alone is, of course, insufficient. Training must be completed by thorough practice of the method. The test is first demonstrated to the candidate, who then executes it, first under close supervision, and later on by himself in parallel to tests done by the instructor. Discrepancies must be recognized, explained and eliminated by further training.

Testing in the ward is generally restricted to physicians and nursing staff. On the other hand a stay at the hospital is an ideal occasion for initiation of self control by a diabetic patient. We may be obliged to simplify the teaching phase of such patients, as they often lack the necessary scientific background, insisting all the more on practice and training, and the importance of recording true results. An important study has shown that patients have a strong tendency to 'optimize' their record.

In addition to teaching and training non-professional users we must convince them that quality control is not a nuisance but certainly a benefit for them and for their patients.

Table 12.4 Teaching programme for the nursing staff.

I. Pre-analytical precautions:
    Preparation of the patient
    Specimen collection
    Specimen handling
    Identification of the patient and the specimen
    Storage

II. Information concerning the analyte:
    Normal and pathological metabolism of the analyte
    Significance of positive or negative reactions, and of high
      or low values
    Degree of emergency of the results
    Consequences

III. Information concerning the analytical procedure:
    Mechanism of the test
    Execution of the test
    Limitations of the test (sensitivity, range, margin of error)
    Interferences
    Stability of the reagents
    Storage of the reagents
    Special precautions

IV. Clerical tasks:
    Transmission of the results
    Storage of the results

Discussion

Martin	What materials can you see us using in the short term for QC?
Kutter	Serum analyses present no problem as lots of materials are available. The situation is more complicated as far as urine in concerned. For example urobilinogen is very unstable even in the frozen state unless ascorbate is added - but this interferes with glucose assays. Concentrations of analytes should be around physiological levels and not very high.
Netter	You have described control in wards but what about control by the private practitioner who can only use manufacturers products. I suggest that the only possibility for him would be to get in touch with a central laboratory.
Kutter	Serum is no problem but whole blood presents difficulties.
Dybkaer	We accept that all results should be checked by quality control. In the central laboratory this does not present a problem since adequate statistical procedures can be set up using large pools of material. For decentralized instruments we need a different statistical approach if we are not to overburden the patient.
Kutter	This is also a very costly problem. Ideally quality control should be carried out every time an instrument is used. However the patient's quality control specimens may be kept in a hot car or under some equally unsatisfactory storage conditions making the material unsuitable for long term use.
Calam	Why not include a temperature indicating strip with each set of reagents. The WHO uses this approach when supplying vaccines to tropical countries.

13

Special Considerations in Haematology and Blood Banking

Deryk W Dawson

BASIC CONSIDERATIONS

Decentralization in haematology is still minimal and the particular problems relating to the speciality are only just beginning to appear. Certain questions need consideration before the appropriate standards can be formulated because different answers will indicate different requirements.

Why does the test need doing outside the department?

Presumably it will be for the patients' benefit - it is unlikely to be economic even if large numbers of simple tests are done which require no central laboratory back-up. For example, haemoglobin screening of well populations in developed countries has never been shown to be of benefit either for the individual or for the community.

Where are the tests to be done?

The standards required in a clinic, acute unit or operating theatre may be different from those needed in a small hospital with a satellite 'hot' laboratory. In the former the repertoire will be smaller and their accuracy could be less than in the latter.

What sorts of tests may be required?

They may be screening procedures, which could require confirmatory tests later (the likely tests for clinical units), or definitive (as in the satellite laboratory). They may be routine but more effectively done at the bedside, urgent because of the clinical situation or required on site because the main laboratory is closed.

Who will do the tests?

Will it be a doctor, nurse, pharmacist or someone attached to the unit for this specific purpose? The turnover of junior medical staff is such that their training and supervision would be a constant and demanding work-load on the central laboratory. Nursing administration on the other hand may expect to train their own staff rather than involve the laboratory, an expectation which should be resisted. In some situations it may be more effective to allot laboratory staff to do the decentralized tests, e.g. in antenatal and anticoagulant clinics.

MAINTAINING ANALYTICAL QUALITY

Two general principles for good performance of any test should be applied to decentralized ones - quality assurance, both internal and external, and the standardization of methods. But as important as written and material standards would be early and continuing liaison between the main department and the clinician in regard to purchase and use of equipment, compliance with health and safety regulations and the training of the staff of the unit. Tests in satellite laboratories should be done by staff seconded from the main laboratory. It may be remembered that centralization occurred not only because of the introduction of expensive multichannel analysers but also because the standard of performance in satellite laboratories infrequently approached that of the main laboratory unless there was interchange of staff.

SPECIFIC CONSIDERATIONS IN HAEMATOLOGY

There are few haematology tests at present suitable for decentralization to areas other than to small laboratories though developments in technology are likely to expand the range. Particular points in regard to some haematology tests, which may affect the writing of standards are as follows.

Haemoglobin
The quality of performance required will depend on its purpose. In an antenatal clinic, for example, where more than one measurement over a period to time on each patient will be required, as high a standard of accuracy as in the main laboratory will be required, whereas in an acute unit such accuracy will not be necessary since

only gross differences in haemoglobin would be significant. In some sites (e.g. antenatal clinics) haemoglobin without mean corpuscular volume (MCV) may be inadequate. It is unfortunate that at least one haemoglobinometer suitable for general use will take the user back to archaic percentage units. On the other hand it is the only haematology measurement for which there are both national and international material standards.

Haematocrit
The accuracy of this measurement should be the same wherever the test is done.

Leukocyte count
The accuracy should be similar to that in the central laboratory but the cost of equipment would be high for an individual unit though reasonable for a satellite laboratory. An abnormal count without differential may be adequate for an out-patient department following patient progress but would not always be satisfactory for an emergency area, where simple two-cell differentials, distinguishing neutrophils from other leukocytes, and platelet counts in microhaematocrit tubes may be sufficient.

Erythrocyte sedimentation rate (ESR)
This began in most hospitals as a ward test and could beneficially return there. An advantage is the ICSH (International Committee for Standardization in Haematology) reference method though there is no standard or reference material.

Haemoglobinopathies
There is a need for urgent testing for Haemoglobin S in casualty departments, theatres, dental departments, etc., though the present technology has limitations of which many present non-laboratory users are unaware. Nor is there general appreciation that the test is a screening procedure which always requires confirmation by electrophoresis. Glucose-6-phosphate dehydrogenase screening techniques are unsatisfactory. However the need for urgent estimations has been overstated.

Coagulation tests
The prothrombin time (ratio) is already done in many anticoagulant clinics though it is usually performed by laboratory staff. This is appropriate if clinics are at a distance from the laboratory and a large number of patients are to be seen. Other tests upon which patient management may depend, e.g. the control of fibrinolytic and heparin therapy, could be done with benefit at the bedside. The detection of fibrinogen/fibrin degradation products is a suitably devolved test, though without other investigations, which require laboratory involvement, the result is of limited value.

Blood transfusion
This must be the most debatable area. ABO grouping could be done on site or in the ambulance to save time in obtaining appropriate blood. Patients who have been grouped and screened for antibodies of clinical significance may be candidates for a simple ABO compatability test in the theatre or acute unit. This practice would reduce some of the present potential documentation errors. However, blood would also have to be available on site and blood banking procedures (refrigerator maintenance, stock-keeping, etc.) would have to be introduced.

Workload and costs
The effect of decentralization on the laboratory also requires consideration. It is unlikely that the resiting of tests will reduce the laboratory workload for some time. Initially overall health service costs will increase because of both the additional tests and the additional responsibilities placed upon the central laboratory.

CONCLUSIONS

Because the situation ahead will differ from site to site, reference both to degrees of accuracy and precision required and to particular analyses, except as examples, should be avoided in written guidelines. Only blood banking, with its therapeutic component and health agency regulations, calls for specific instructions. Written standards for decentralized haematology tests should therefore be general guidelines capable of application to both present and future tests, to tests done in both clinical units and satellite laboratories and to tests performed by a variety of individuals with minimal scientific training.

Discussion

Stewart   You stated that costs would increase with decentralized testing. Which costs have you considered?

Dawson   We have only considered laboratory costs but have not taken into account savings in patient time, travel etc. These are very difficult to assess.

14

Special Considerations in Histopathology and Cytology

Nils Stormby

HISTOPATHOLOGY

Histopathology is based on the microscopical examination of tissue sections from surgical specimens, be they small biopsies or large and complex organ resectates, as for example the result of a Wertheim operation. In many respects histopathology assures the quality of other laboratory methods by confirming the presence of a tumour and more specifically the type of it. Although histopathology is one of the oldest disciplines in medicine, it has been closely following the developments in molecular biology and immunology with the introduction of such methods as DNA measurements and immunohistochemistry etc. Due to the vast base of knowledge in histopathology there has also been a need for extensive subspecializations.

Histopathological examination plays a decisive role in many diseases with a focus on tumours. The diagnostic results are highly individual-related and demand not only knowledge and experience but also a mental stability due to the trace of subjectivity which exists in the type of examinations where patterns are judged and not measured. Quality assurance is therefore mandatory in histopathology as many clinicians and unfortunately many pathologists regard the histological findings as the difinitive result. Quality assurance in histopathology requires a continuous feedback of clinical data and a follow-up when possible on the autopsy table.

CYTOLOGY

Cytology, almost exclusively for cancer detection, is based on examinations of cells only and diagnostic conclusions are drawn from such details as the form and shape of the cytoplasm and nucleus, the nucleolus etc. In a cytological smear it is impossible to appreciate one of the general criteria of malignant disease, namely the invasive pattern and from this point of view it is actually not possible in sensu strictu to make a diagnosis of malignancy. From the cells one can conclude only that they are originating from carcinoma.

Cytology has two branches: one is named exfoliative cytology where cells from mucosal linings are scraped off and smeared onto glass slides. Cells from various normal or pathological body fluids can also be collected, concentrated and smeared. The other branch is fine needle aspiration cytology, a method based on cellular material achieved by needling palpable lesions or lesions visualized by X-ray, ultrasound etc in inner organs. The diagnosis is based on the same principles as in exfoliative cytology.

ORGANIZATIONAL CONSIDERATIONS

It is clear that cytology has its base in histopathology both as a source of knowledge and for methods of quality assurance. Therefore there is a need of close cooperation preferably by keeping the disciplines tightly together in the same premises or at least organization and backed up by an integrated computer system retrieving earlier diagnostic information, both cytological and histopathological, in the individual case. This can be well illustrated with precancer and cancer of the uterine cervix, where lesions are primarily diagnosed by cytology and later confirmed (and even cured) by colposcopically directed biopsies which are taken for histopathological examination. It is not uncommon that the different diagnostic approaches in these cases give different initial results which require not only new sections from the tissue blocks, rescreening of smears etc but also an organization designed for such retrievals.

It is therefore obvious that both histopathology and exfoliative cytology are best organized together. Furthermore a laboratory organization has to be of a certain size to be cost-efficient and as in cytology to assure quality. Thus, it is doubtful if a yearly number of histopathological specimens below 5,000 is acceptable - when it comes to cytology no less than 10,000 gynecological smears and 1,500 other exfoliative specimen are necessary. These figures indicate that a decentralization of services will not improve, but lower the standards.

One exception, however, is fine needle aspiration cytology. The technique is simple and harmless to the patient and a smear from the needle aspirate from for example a tumour of the neck can be processed in a few minutes and give a firm diagnosis of a benign cyst, a lymphoadenosis, a cancer metastasis etc. However, although the needling is easy the technique must be thoroughly practiced to ensure that the target is correctly hit and the smearing of the aspirate perfect. Moreover, the diagnostic work is a job for the superspecialist, well trained and experienced in histopathology. Who shall perform the needling and where it shall be made is under continuous dispute but it is for sure that this wonderful method can never be the instrument for everybody. Optimal results are obtained when the cytologist himself examines and needles the patient. On the other hand when various clinicians take specimens between 25-50% of the smears in various series are so poor that no diagnostic conclusion can be made, thus speaking against a decentralized service.

Discussion

Boroviczény   Much of what you say comes from my own heart. In haematology we need both centralization and decentralization but we must have quality control. I once sent out my own marrow for histological opinion. I found that in the opinion of my colleagues I had many serious diseases but now many years later I am still alive. We have kept on doing experiments like this and find we are getting better.

Killander   Specimens must be sent out around the world to compare histological opinions. What sort of results are found?

Stormby   I participated in such a survey in the USA and we decided that the results were too dangerous to publish because of a considerable disagreement. We have repeated the exercises and are now seeing some improvement.

15

Organization and Management in the Decentralized Laboratory

Robert M Rowan

INTRODUCTION

Management is defined as the organization of a properly functioning enterprise to achieve defined goals. In many ways the problems of organization and management in the decentralized laboratory constitute a relatively simple topic to deal with, certainly at a theoretical level. The problems arising do not differ qualitatively from those in the large centralized laboratory: they differ only in a matter of scale. In both instances the aim is to deliver the correct result for the appropriate patient at the right time. Some may say that this approach is naive but are they justified in such an assertion? In both centralized and decentralized laboratories, one is, after all, dealing with patient samples, technical operators, technical methods, quality control, laboratory results and their interpretation.

What is meant by a decentralized laboratory? The areas which must be considered are:

(1) Small laboratories which are within the confines of a hospital but which are neither attached administratively to main laboratories nor subject to the same regulatory forces, e.g. research laboratories attached to clinical departments which have evolved to give a service output.

(2) Laboratories in high utility clinical areas, e.g. intensive care etc., which have evolved outwith the administrative and regulatory control of centralized laboratories.

(3) Ward side-rooms and ward bedside testing.

(4) Laboratories in the physician's office.

(5)   Testing in the patient's home and patient self-monitoring.

(6)   A special case may be made for the multi-disciplinary laboratory in a small hospital, e.g. a private institution, in which medical, scientific and technical staff have not been trained in each of the disciplines represented.

Guidelines for laboratory practice should be available for use in such areas to ensure validity of the technology employed, correct application of this technology, quality of result, training and safety of personnel.

IS THERE A REQUIREMENT FOR DECENTRALIZATION?

The factors which determine the need for decentralization are several. Perhaps the most important is the clinical requirement for immediate results. This may be so because of the urgency of a clinical situation or for the convenience of the physician or of the patient. Technical complexity of testing is an important limiting factor and automation is not necessarily an answer to this since most automated instruments require considerable technical expertise to keep them operating properly. Comparative costs of centralized and decentralized testing must also enter into the equation. On the less attractive side, the profit motive is a powerful incentive. The cynic will say that this is the only real justification for decentralization and may be the only reason for its perpetuation.

Historically, laboratory testing was carried out close to the patient. Increase in the number of available procedures and the development of automated instruments led inexorably to the centralization of laboratory facilities. A move is now afoot by clinicians to revive side-room diagnostic testing, and this is aided and abetted by a proliferation of small, portable, comparatively inexpensive instruments produced by manufacturers who have been quick to appreciate that a market exists. What must not be forgotten is that these instruments perform laboratory analyses and the only persons capable of rational evaluation of these tests, the technology and the economics are workers trained in laboratory practices.

THE CONCEPT OF MANAGEMENT GUIDELINES

The concepts to be embodied in appropriate guidelines can be summarized under three headings, namely management, operation and finance. Management concepts are subdivided into planning and responsibility for organization, staffing, direction and supervision.

Pre-eminent amongst management tasks is planning. As in all laboratory operations, planning is critical. As Goethe said, 'to plan and not act is futile; to act and not plan is fatal'. Planning may be

defined as the methodical and logical selection of a series of com-
plementary actions for the purpose of pursuing and achieving an
objective. Central to this is an understanding not only of existing
but of future requirements, of current circumstances and, most
importantly, of current limitations. In this respect the decentralized facility may differ radically from the large centralized
laboratory. In the latter the existing professional environment ensures that personnel are trained to the highest standards of
laboratory medicine. This may not be the case in the small
laboratory and certainly will not be the case in the clinical side-
room nor in the physician's office where other skills are the rule.
Every person associated with laboratory testing must recognize that
identification, documentation and accomplishment of meaningful and
realistic objectives are of major importance to correct laboratory
practice. Association with and advice from a larger laboratory
should ensure the correct planning approach in the decentralized
laboratory.

OPERATIONAL PLANNING FOR DECENTRALIZED TESTING

Operation is defined as the sum of the different activities involved
in any enterprise. Operational data essential for laboratory planning include:

(1)   Previous experience: This is perhaps the most important of
      all organisational resources.

(2)   Clinical requirement.

(3)   Competence: Can the decentralized laboratory perform a test
      more quickly and with the same accuracy as the central
      laboratory?

(4)   Physician/laboratory relationships: Many of the problems in
      this respect can be attributed to the less than full and
      mutual appreciation of the difficulties which the other group
      has. An element of decentralization can often go a long way
      to resolve such problems.

(5)   Regulatory and accrediting forces: No one should argue
      against well-conceived and realistic standards by which the
      quality of performance in any laboratory can be objectively
      measured.

(6)   Trends: These serve as valuable indicators of consensus
      thinking and may support or reverse personal persuasion and
      anticipation. Trends are, however, not always based on valid
      assumptions nor are they always of long duration.

THE PATIENT AND DECENTRALIZED TESTING

It is against this background that guidelines for management and organization in decentralized laboratory testing must be constructed. Such guidelines must be comprehensive, unambiguous and subject to regular review. The following topics must be addressed specifically.

SPECIFIC CONSIDERATIONS

Definition of responsibilities

This is a three-tiered operation. Administrative responsibility includes the definition of job specifications and job descriptions. It is important to appreciate that these differ. The job specification is designed to protect management and defines those requirements, both professional and personal, which best suits an individual for a given job. The job description, on the other hand, is designed to protect the employee and defines those tasks which an individual in employment is expected to perform. Also included under the heading of administrative responsibility is the creation of work schedules to deal with an anticipated workload. Personnel must be available when work requires to be done but since staff accounts for the largest component of cost in any operation, strenuous efforts must be made to ensure their most effective utilization. Particular attention must be paid to any requirement for emergency duties. Technical responsibility includes the distribution of duties, ensuring adequate performance standards of testing, the supervision of laboratory work, the supervision of quality control procedures and communication procedures. Finally, the hierarchical structure must be defined with clear delegation of responsibilities, compliance with statutory and legal regulations and for trade union affairs.

Availability of facilities

These constitute important responsibilities of management and will differ depending on location of testing. Clearly the requirements in the physician's office are very different from those in the small multidisciplinary laboratory, but minimum requirements must be defined for each. In general, facilities must be sufficient to permit the performance of a test with defined precision and accuracy and without endangering the operator or any third party. In the interests of patient and staff safety the laboratory should be divided into three procedural zones for venesection, laboratory testing and administration. Facilities to be considered include such items as space, services, furnishings, equipment and materials. It is important to remember that instruments may have a requirement for environmental control, special electricity supply and plumbing. Choice of tests and equipment will be determined by clinical requirements, the volume of requests anticipated, the margins of error which are tolerable, the degree of urgency, the ease of maintenance, the availability of servicing and spare parts and by the availability, cost and shelf-life of reagents. Although perhaps difficult to achieve, recommended methods shoud be defined for each circumstance. Choice should not be determined by the eloquence of sales representatives alone.

Availability of qualified personnel

What qualifications are required for the performance of a particular task? These will be determined by the need for manual technical skills, for expertise with instruments and, of course, ultimately on test complexity. A spectrum of individuals will be available but obviously not all will be suitable in each location. This spectrum will range over:

(1)　The specially trained nurse;

(2)　The laboratory aide, an individual trained in a narrow range of simple repetitive practical skills but with little emphasis on theoretical scientific instruction;

(3)　The laboratory technologist with nationally acceptable qualifications by which his skills may be quantified;

(4)　The medical practitioner with relevant practical training in a limited range of simple tests; and

(5)　The medical practitioner with specialist laboratory training in one or more disciplines of laboratory medicine.

Clear recognition of the training required for specific tests in different locations must be written into all guideline documents.

Training of personnel

While minimal training requirements will be defined in the job description, specific and continuing education of all personnel is necessary and can be achieved in a variety of ways. Training to carry out existing procedures may be carried out on site. For the introduction of improved or new methods training may be obtained at reference laboratories or at courses conducted by industry, professional societies or government agencies. A requirement for continuing education should be written into job descriptions.

Provision of standard operating procedures

These should include procedures not only for sample handling, technical methods, preventive maintenance, quality control and issue of results, but also for safety procedures for the protection of staff against accident by physical or chemical agents and infection from samples. Obviously hepatitis B and HIV infections are particularly important but basic rules for laboratory hygiene should not be neglected. Careful use should be made of any national guidelines documents when establishing laboratory codes of practice. Good laboratory practice dictates that operating procedures should be in writing and that such documents be given to all employees who then sign as having read and understood them. Ensuring compliance with operating procedures is an important supervisory task. Only procedures which have been found applicable in practice should be recommended in any decentralized location.

Reporting of results

This is the end-product of the laboratory procedure without which the laboratory cannot achieve its goal in patient care. It is appropriate, therefore, that due attention is paid to this. Not only must the test result be clear and unequivocal, but the report format must also be designed in such a way that it is compatible with other patient records. For a variety of reasons laboratory records must be kept but it is a matter for debate as to how long these records should be maintained. It is important to appreciate that just like the patient's case-notes, laboratory results are confidential, and arrangements must be made to ensure their confidentiality. Clear lines for communicating results from laboratory worker to clinician must also be defined.

Quality control

This is a programme for assuring reliability of result. It falls naturally into two components namely non-analytical quality control and analytical quality control. The former includes request specifications, worksheets, specimen collection equipment, patient identification details, container identification, delivery of specimens, storage of specimens, handling and separation of specimens and distribution of results. These should all be specified in writing. Analytical quality control functions include method reliability, instrument calibration, reagent quality and the testing of biological controls. This last aspect of quality control is widely recognized and is further subdivided into internal quality control and external quality assessment. There is universal agreement that both are mandatory for the correct performance of any laboratory test.

Inventory management

The procurement of laboratory supplies is greatly facilitated by an inventory system which identifies all supply needs and the quantity of items to be kept immediately available. The system must allow personnel both a means of identifying depletions and a means for triggering timely replacement. It must be closely monitored, regularly updated and kept sufficiently flexible to permit change. Provision of an appropriate storage environment is an important concept in inventory control as is a scheme for use of products in chronological order within their specified shelf-lives. Responsibilities for these functions must be clearly defined.

Purchasing and service contracts

All laboratory activities incur expense. However in every case such expenditure may be controlled to some extent. Continuous efforts must be made to attain the most effective balance between quality and cost of services. Cost control is the means by which such a balance is maintained. Quality at any price is unrealistic and must be substituted by the practice of cost-effectiveness. As a generalization, choice of product is determined by the existence of an acceptable evaluation by competent authority, the guarantee of regular availability of supplies and the availability of comprehensive maintenance contracts where applicable. The importance of service contracts cannot be overestimated for the following reasons. First, they contribute to cost savings by prolonging the lives of instruments, and additionally they result in the diminution of 'down time'. Secondly, such maintenance of instruments contributes to overall quality control. Finally, any practice which reduces equipment malfunction with its attendant hazards contributes to the safety and well-being of laboratory workers. Service contracts must specify the exact nature of the service in a detailed 'who pays for what' manner. Factors which invalidate a service contract should also be clearly identified. Leasing as opposed to purchase of an item of equipment may be explored.

Budgeting

The term 'budgeting' implies a scarcity of financial resource.

(1) Capital/revenue budgeting: There are two forms of budgeting: (a) capital budgeting is the process of planning the spending of capital for new projects to yield long-term benefits; and (b) revenue or operations budgeting is the process of allocating limited resources to maintaining existing projects.
        Although accountancy problems are best dealt with by

professional accountants, some knowledge of the principles involved is very necessary. Capital expenditure should be regarded as an investment; at worst it should 'break even' but at best it should result in profit. As with any potential investment, rate of return on capital should be evaluated and used as a criterion for budgeting decisions. Allied to this are justification and priority of need. Four justification categories exist, namely (a) replacement of equipment beyond repair, (b) increased workload, (c) cost reduction, and (d) new and/or improved technology.

(2)   <u>Records of transaction:</u>   A good record system is essential for the management of income as well as costs. Payments by patients and all other agencies must be carefully recorded. On the cost side, salaries, rentals, taxes, services, reagents and all other recurring expenses must be meticulously noted.

(3)   <u>Price fixing:</u>   Correct pricing is not obtained by guess work nor should it be obtained by matching with another laboratory's price. It must have a basis in logic and fact. This becomes particularly relevant in the event of third party request, whether by government agency or consumer group, for explanation of widely differing or exorbitantly high prices.

CONCLUSIONS

It has to be conceded that laboratory practice has now evolved from a service unit into a business entity. It is no longer sufficient to be technically competent and scientifically innovative. Financial resources are limited while costs relentlessly increase. The laboratory must, therefore, frequently justify its financial needs, account for its performance and be seen to be a safe place in which to work. This is a logical and correct approach. The centralized laboratory has been moving towards these goals for some years. Such principles must apply equally to the decentralized laboratory. The provision of topic guidelines should aid this process. These guidelines must be comprehensive but above all they must be realistic.

Discussion

Shinton   Could you say a little more about the relationship between the centralized and decentralized laboratory in ideal circumstances?

Rowan Ideally they should be related, with the central laboratory playing a major role. But then the decentralized laboratory becomes a satellite laboratory. GPs need a lot of help.

Calam We should not ignore the pharmacist. In the UK they offer a good service for pregnancy testing and have good quality control. They could be much more important in other countries. Should reimbursement be offered to all pharmacies? Dr Dybkaer's committees might take this area into account.

Kirkemo The clinical laboratory produces a product but who is the customer? Is it the patient, the clinician or the patient's family? We can never win an argument with a customer until we know who he is. In making any recommendations we must understand the customer and what he wants.

Rowan The doctor patient relationship is paramount and we cannot change this. Other consultative mechanisms must be ancillary to that.

Christensen We have talked about administration etc. but not the product. Who should collect all the data? Should this be the central laboratory?

Rowan Any laboratory which generates data must be responsible for its own record system. Even patients who self test must be responsible.

Stewart As a health service administrator may I ask to whom these guidelines should be addressed? Main laboratories and their satellites would be covered by Dr Leijnse's code of practice but every other laboratory not responsible to a central laboratory should be offered guidelines.

Dybkaer Main laboratories would be covered by the code of practice to be produced by Dr Leijnse's committee. The Standing Action Committee should not get diverted from its main task of producing something for decentralized testing.

Leighton There is good evidence from published quality control data that central laboratories cannot control their own satellites. Therefore how can they be expected to control decentralized laboratories, GP practices etc. They have not got the resources to tackle this problem.

Jennings In the UK we are looking at other ways in which this can be done. There may be alternatives to the central laboratories. Furthermore as instruments continue to develop they may become self-controlling.

Tryding   It is important not to use the word 'control' outside the central laboratory. For psychological reasons we should use the term 'quality assurance'.

Mill   The question of how resources are provided is not the major issue. The role of the ECCLS is to provide a standard and this can then be used as ammunition by individual countries in their fights for funding.

Calam   Clinical usefulness is most important. If doctors office testing is clinically useful then quality control will naturally follow. Also the importance of legal sanction must not be underestimated. If a manufacturer provided a kit which gave an incorrect result which in turn led to an inappropriate clinical decision, legal action might be taken. This may be an important regulatory factor.

Part 5

COST IMPLICATIONS OF DECENTRALIZED TESTING

16

Cost Implications of Decentralized Testing – A Health Agency's View

Robert Netter

Europe does not yet have a unified approach to decentralized testing, and nor does France itself. The views presented in this paper are therefore personal.

THE PRESENT SITUATION

Decentralized testing is not new in France and has been carried out in side wards for a long time. However national authorities are no longer encouraging this for both technical and economic reasons. As in the UK, pharmacists are authorized to carry out some simple tests. A list of approved tests is presently being defined by the authorities and these will be reimbursed by social security if requested by a physician. In the emergency situation non-biologists are also performing some tests. These procedures include confirmatory tests for blood grouping and blood gas analysis during surgery, transportation of critically ill patients and the surveillance of premature babies.

Other examples of decentralized testing include the determination of alcohol by policemen at the roadside and home testing. In the latter case the cost of reagents is not reimbursed by social security except for glucose testing materials which are prescribed by a physician.

JURIDICAL ASPECTS

1. Only biologists who have received special training are allowed to practise clinical testing and be reimbursed by social security, with some exceptions clearly defined by the law.

2.   Self-prescription of minor drugs is quite common and, in the absence of any reimbursement, the same could apply to laboratory tests without their being considered illegal practices.

3.   Tests carried out by doctors are tolerated if they do not generate new expenses.

RECOMMENDATIONS

1.   Home tests should be reliable and cheap, and give clear results.

2.   A false negative result due to lack of sensitivity is probably more important than a false positive, because in the latter case a correct result will be obtained when the user contacts either a biologist for confirmation of the result or a clinician for appropriate treatment. On the other hand excessive sensitivity may generate increased numbers of other costly determinations.

3.   Doctor's testing should not require heavy equipment or high technology.

4.   Great care should be taken with information for users if the test requires interpretation. It seems hazardous to put a reagent for AIDS diagnosis only on the market, as gonorrhoea, syphilis and hepatitis B should also be considered in these patients.

5.   The handling of infectious specimens by people not acquainted with good laboratory practice might be hazardous.

6.   The same quality should be required whether reagents are used in centralized or decentralized laboratories or for home tests (reproducibility, sensitivity, specificity and stability). The same reagent or apparatus may be used in both situations but the main difference is that the people carrying out the tests have not received the same level of training. Also, doctor's tests are less likely to be accompanied by a positive or negative control although quality assessment is considered essential for clinical laboratories. With the help of scientific societies, it should be possible to adapt such quality assurance systems for testing by doctors. However, it will be more difficult to adopt similar systems for home tests except for some routine assays such as glucose determinations.

ECONOMIC ASPECTS

(1)   Laboratory centralization was considered to be more economical for a long time but this situation might change with the simplification of some tests.

(2)   In France it is difficult to make cost/benefit analyses of home and doctors' tests as only those performed by biologists are reimbursed.

(3)   For home pregnancy testing, which is not reimbursed by social security, the expense for the patient is higher than if the test was performed by a clinical laboratory. Moreover the marketing of such reagents has not reduced the number of tests performed by clinical laboratories.

(4)   The absence of reimbursement for doctors' testing limits not only the expenses for the national authorities but also the development of such tests.

CONCLUSIONS

Two main tendencies are apparent. The first is the centralization of some tests requiring costly machinery or high technology. The second is towards decentralization, pregnancy testing by immunoenzymatic methods being a good example.

Such simplification encourages routine testing which, as in the case of blood in faeces, could be carried out free of charge as a home test. However, national authorities should be aware that due to the extreme sensitivity of this particular test there could be a consequent increase in the numbers of other costly determinations.

In the promotion of home and doctors' tests, speed is recognized as an important factor. However in the absence of external quality assessment these tests can be considered only as 'presumptive tests'.

Discussion

Rowan	You mentioned that there should be consideration of tests for decentralization by the national authority. Is this in terms of vetting the types of tests as suitable for decentralization?
Netter	In France we have an agreement for decentralized glucose testing. We say that

this can be done at home. In the future other tests of importance could be discussed for reimbursement but each case must be considered on its merits.

17

Cost Implications of Decentralized Testing – A Laboratorian's View

Rainer Haeckel

INTRODUCTION

In the last decade a worldwide trend away from decentralized laboratory services towards central units has been observed in most larger hospitals. While it has been generally believed that centralization considerably improves the overall efficiency, the development of new technologies has recently brought the possibility of decentralization to the forefront of scientific discussion. Clinical chemists must therefore reassess whether centralization provides the efficiency expected.

The efficiency of centralized laboratory services is expected to be superior to that of the decentralized situation in several areas including data handling, analytical spectrum, expertise, emergency services, economics and timing. This paper presents some thoughts on the economic aspects of decentralized testing nearer the patient. So far no data has been published from any cost study which could be used to discuss this topic, and therefore two typical situations have been chosen for a cost comparison to be made.

COST COMPARISONS OF CENTRALIZED VS. DECENTRALIZED TESTING

A problem-oriented cost analysis study was performed, neglecting all costs which would have been identical for all alternatives and considering only those costs which were relevant for the comparison purpose. It must therefore be emphasized that the costs shown below do not represent total costs for any particular activity.

The ECCLS subcommittee on cost analysis has prepared recommendations for such a problem-oriented cost comparison. These recommendations are followed in the present study and the same nomenclature is used. Costs for personnel are considered as effective working time as suggested by a joint working group of the Austrian and German Society for Clinical Chemistry (Figure 17.1).

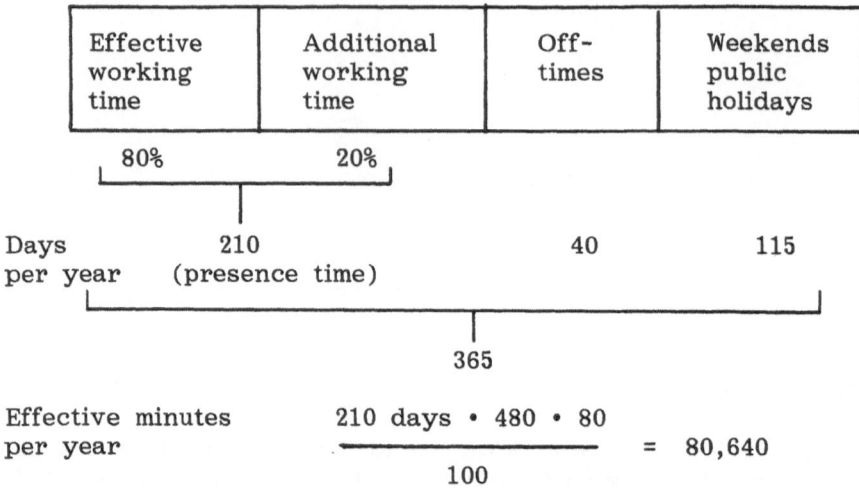

Figure 17.1 Calculation of the effective minutes per year assuming that the average year has 365 days and the official daily working time is 480 minutes.

Alternative approaches to glucose testing

In the first example the costs for determination of blood glucose concentration are studied assuming a daily workload of about 400 tests. Three alternatives are compared.

In **alternative I** all tests are performed in a centralized unit using one analyser (e.g. an Eppendorf ACP 5040), one technician and a kinetic hexokinase method on haemolysed capillary blood specimens.

In **alternative II** 90% of all tests are performed as in the first alternative and 10% are performed at the bedside (e.g. in an emergency ward or in a diabetic unit) using a test strip procedure with reflectometric measurement (Reflocheck system).

In **alternative III** 50% of all tests are performed as in the first alternative and 50% with a Reflocheck system. In this case 10 reflectometers are required in 10 units. The various types of costs are specified in detail in Table 17.1. All costs are presented in German Marks (1985/86).

COST IMPLICATIONS - A LABORATORIANS'S VIEW

Table 17.1 **A breakdown** of the cost of glucose estimations

	ACP 5040			REFLOLUX II	
Number of tests:	400	360	200	200	40
Number of analysers:	1	1	1	10	1
Capital costs	123,799			5,392	539
(purchase price)					
Annual depreciation	19,189			932	93
(interest rate:6%)					
Life time (years)	8			8	
Working days per year	250			250	
Disposables per test	0.06			0.02	
Additional fixed costs per batch*	8			-	
Service costs as percentage	5			5	
of capital cost					
Reagents per test	0.11			0.96	
Personnel time per workload (min)				400	80
Cost per effective minute				0.65**	
Personnel cost per day	247.6	247.6	185.7		

* includes the cost of items such as reagents, calibrators, printer paper, lamps
  etc. (2000 DM: 250 days)

** 52,000 DM ÷ (100,800 min per year. 0.8) ≈ 0.65

For alternatives I and II it is assumed that one technician is required in the central unit to perform a daily workload of 400 tests. The total costs for one technician are about 243 DM per day. In alternative III, 60% of the technician's capacity is used. For the Reflolux the estimated time for one test is 2 minutes. Times for quality control and maintenance are not considered. Furthermore, sampling and data handling time on the ward have been neglected because they are probably identical in all alternatives. The fixed and variable cost for the various alternatives are summed up in Table 17.2. These costs divided by the number of tests give the cost per test which is then used to calculate the cost of the 400 tests for the three alternatives.

Table 17.3 clearly demonstrates that decentralization leads to a cost increase for laboratory services in larger hospitals. Even if labour costs on the ward are neglected, the costs of alternatives II and III are 460 and 532 DM respectively in comparison to 427 DM for alternative I. The glucose test has been chosen as a commonly used example but similar conclusions may be drawn with other analytes.

111

Table 17.2 Fixed and variable costs (DM) for glucose estimations

	ACP 5040			REFLOLUX II	
Number of tests	400	360	200	200	40
Number of analysers	1	1	1	10	1
Fixed costs per batch	111.6	111.6	111.6	4.5	0.45
Variable costs per batch	315.6	308.8	219.7	456	91.2
Fixed plus variable costs	427	420	331.3	460.5	91.7
Costs per test	1.06	1.16	1.64	2.30	2.29

Table 17.3 Total cost (DM) of glucose estimations in three different laboratory configurations

	Alternative I	Alternative II	Alternative III
Number of tests per day in central unit (ACP 5040)	400	360	200
Number of tests per day in one decentralized unit	0	40	0
Number of tests per day in ten decentralized units	0	0	200
Costs of 400 tests	427	512	792

Organization of emergency testing

In the second example emergency testing in a central unit is compared with emergency testing in three decentralized units in a large hospital.

Alternative A represents a central emergency laboratory which is operated independently from other routine sections of a central laboratory. Two technicians run the night shift. The instrumentation may be on average two years old (Table 17.4).

Table 17.4   **Instrumentation used in alternative A**

Instrument	Actual costs[1]
1 Multitest analyser (G400)	204,050
1 Coagulometer (4 channels)	4,064
2 Microscopes	15,668
1 Sysmex CC 700	94,129
2 Blood gas analysers (ABL 3)	76,892
1 Thrombocounter	31,339
1 Centrifuge (Labofuge)	4,897
1 Centrifuge (Biofuge)	1,178
1 Spectrometer (Eppendorf PCP)	22,662
1 Singletest analyser (ACP 5040)	144,250
Total	599,129

[1] All costs are in DM, including accessories and VAT (1983).

For **alternative B** the following assumptions have been made:

- At least three satellite units are required, one of these replacing the present emergency laboratory. The latter remains as a central unit to which the technicians always return after a request has been completed in one of the other units. The central unit is situated in the department of internal medicine close to the emergency ward. Another unit would be placed in the emergency ward of the paediatric department and the third unit in the department of surgery.

- In the satellite units only a small set of emergency tests should be performed: blood gas analysis, the determination of glucose, creatinine and/or urea, some electrolytes, coagulation tests, haemoglobin, and the counting of leukocytes, erythrocytes and thrombocytes. Less urgent analyses should

113

be performed after the technician has returned to the central unit.

- For both alternatives the same number of personnel are required and therefore personnel costs can be neglected. In alternative B less staff are needed for the transport of specimens from the wards to the central laboratory unit. However this cost saving is probably offset by the additional technical staff which may be required by alternative B.

- The configuration of the analytical systems in alternative B was chosen taking into account their speed and cost (Table 17.5). For the clinical chemical analyses a dry-chemistry system which can use whole blood directly was chosen.

- The cost comparison study neglects all problems which may be encountered with chemistry on dry reagent carriers. These primarily concern their poorer specificity and the lack of quality control materials suited to this new technology. It is assumed that these problems will be solved, and that the new techniques will provide acceptable results with patients' specimens.

Table 17.5 Instrumentation used in alternative B

Unit I (Internal Medicine)		Unit II (Surgery)		Unit III (Paediatrics)	
Instrument	Cost	Instrument	Cost	Instrument	Cost
3 Reflotrons	23,940	3 Reflotrons	23,940	1 Reflotron	7,980
1 Coagulometer (4 channels)	4,064	1 Coagulometer (4 channels)	4,064	1 Coagulometer (2 channels)	2,850
1 Microscope	7,834	1 Microscope	7,834	1 Microscope	7,834
1 Sysmex 180	56,202	1 Sysmex 180	56,202	1 Sysmex 150	28,500
1 ABL 3	38,446	1 ABL 3	38,446	1 ABL 3	38,446
1 Labofuge	4,897	1 Labofuge	4,897	1 Labofuge	4,897
1 Biofuge	1,178	-		1 Biofuge	1,178
1 ACP 5040	144,250	-		-	
1 PCP	22,662	-		-	
Total	303,473		135,383		91,685

All costs are in DM, including accessories and VAT (1983/1984)

COST IMPLICATIONS - A LABORATORIANS'S VIEW

In Table 17.6 the costs for the two alternatives are presented. The costs for alternative A were taken from our hospital's computerized financial records for 1984, and those for alternative B were calculated using list prices for the same year. The study has been conducted in cooperation with Boehringer Mannheim.

The data shows that satellite units are more expensive under the present circumstances. Whether possible advantages of timing can be realized for the benefit of the patient must therefore be investigated. In practice such an investigation can only be performed with pilot examples. If such a benefit can be demonstrated, it is still necessary to discuss whether the benefit justifies the expense. So far the author is not aware that anyone has published or even performed such cost/benefit analyses.

Table 17.6 Comparison of annual costs (DM) for Alternatives A and B

	Alternative A	Alternative B
Fixed costs:		
Technical staff[1]	760,000	760,000
Depreciation[2]	74,891	66,318
Capital costs[3]	47,930	42,443
Cleaning	5,591	5,591
Miscellaneous[4]	119,028	119,028
Variable costs:		
Reagents and consumables		
G 400/Reflotron	79,677	400,000
Others	319,694	319,694
Water, energy	3,810	2,000
Maintenance	49,910	3,000
Total	1,460,531	1,745,074

[1] 17 technicians.   [2] 8 years.   [3] 8% interest.
[4] includes general rates distributed by the administration.
Number of requests in 1984 was 625,355

Besides economic considerations, other factors must be considered in the coordinated decentralization of laboratory services (Table 17.7).

Table 17.7 Advantages and disadvantages of satellite units.

Advantages

1. 'Bedside analyses' remain under the responsibility of laboratory specialists and are performed with reference to the central laboratory.

2. Communication with the ward enables adoption of priorities in the sequence of analyses to be performed.

3. Capillary blood taking by technicians can be more easily carried out.

4. Specimens for blood gas analyses can be immediately processed and, therefore, do not require transport on ice.

Disadvantages

1. Data transfer to a central EDP system from several remote units may be difficult.

2. Supervision of several more or less remote units leads to logistic problems.

3. Communication among technicians (especially between well-trained and less-experienced technicians) may be difficult.

4. There may be interference by physicians with the technician's work.

5. Back-up solutions may be difficult to organize.

6. Formation of several small batches which can be nested into each other is usually improbable.

CONCLUSIONS

Several conclusions can be drawn for the present situation from the considerations presented above:

(1) Centralized emergency services must be efficient and have a rapid turnround time for results.

(2) The ideal solution would be to site the main hospital emergency laboratory within the intensive care unit, or at least close to all intensive care units. This situation, however, is not even realized in newly designed hospitals.

(3) As long as this vision is not realized, satellite units under

the supervision of clinical chemists may be useful only in some selected cases. Such an organization could be called coordinated decentralization, which is quite different from uncoordinated decentralization. In former times several units spread over the various departments of larger hospitals performed test programs in parallel, without any cooperation or coordination.

(4)   At the present time satellite units applying carrier-bound reagents are too expensive to replace conventional procedures with multitest analysers in the centralized emergency laboratory units of large hospitals.

(5)   If the emergency services are to be decentralized into several satellite units, so-called dry-chemistry systems may be more economical than conventional procedures with respect to the single unit. However, several satellite units together are more expensive than one central unit. Decentralization of emergency services therefore cannot be justified on economic grounds.

Discussion

Jennings   Is it likely that if tests are available closer to the patient, the number of tests will go down? For example if a specimen is sent to the laboratory there is a tendency for the clinician to request more tests than he immediately requires.

Haeckel   I feel that numbers may increase initially because of differences between results on the ward and in the central laboratory. They may then reduce to their former number but in the long term I cannot see any reason why tests should go down. In a large hospital I cannot see the place for ward testing on any scale.

Bonini   I am convinced that in large hospitals decentralization will result in a big increase in work. In Italy we have legislation preventing the purchase by clinicians of laboratory equipment without the agreement of the central laboratory.

Part 6

SUMMARY AND CONCLUSIONS

18

The Need for Guidelines for Decentralized Clinical Testing

René Dybkaer

INTRODUCTION

Depicting the organization of clinical laboratory testing on a scale from centralized to decentralized, the pointer has recently moved towards the latter position. This is due to new technological possibilities, changed reimbursement schemes, and a shift in the attitudes of both health care personnel and users.

In view of the energy and money spent on centralization during the previous three to four decades, it is natural that the tribe of laboratorians should regard the new trend askance.

Rather than trying to fight the movement, however, the professions should appreciate the new possibilities offered and enter into a collaboration with patients, administration, health agencies, and industry to optimize the process and product. The ECCLS Conference on Decentralized Clinical Testing is an attempt to that end.

THE PATIENT'S SITUATION

Among the many experts giving evidence at this Conference, the testimony of the patient - in the shape of Mrs Seidenfaden - should be especially studied both because it comes from the customer, who is too seldomly heard, and because it contains aspects that are not usually contemplated by the health personnel (Figure 18.1). Such points include the advantage of home-testing in giving the patient the satisfaction of insight into his or her disease and some responsibility for its treatment. Furthermore, the results are situation-relevant in a sense that cannot be achieved in the hospital setting. The disadvantages comprise considerable costs that seem unfair to the patient, the time consumption, and the psychological burden and physiological risk of self-responsibility.

Home-testing requires education and training of the patient as regards therapy and test equipment and of the health personnel in the mental support of the patient. There is also a need to alter

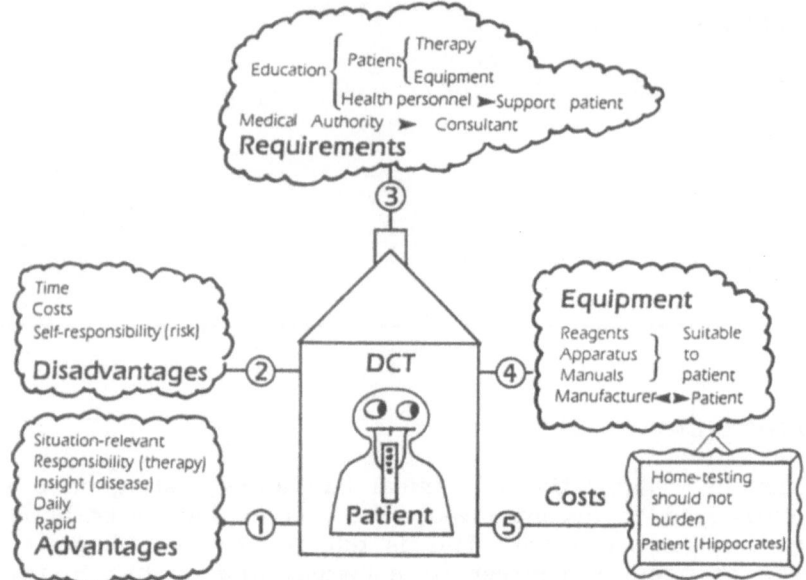

Figure 18.1 Mind map of the patient's relationship to decentralized testing (DCT) in the form of home-testing.

the physician-patient relationship so that the patient regards the physician as a consultant rather than as an authority.

With respect to equipment, the manufacturer should be urged to enter into a dialogue with the patient at an early stage of developing apparatus, reagents, and manuals, as these paraphernalia primarily should suit the patient, rather than the technician.

POSTULATES

Before delineating how the clinical laboratorian could aid the orderly and useful process of decentralization, it is necessary to agree on some assumptions and the following postulates may serve (Figure 18.2):

(1)   The clinical situation determines the required quality of the test result, including analytical and diagnostic characteristics as well as availability and production time of the answer.

(2)   The required quality is independent of the site of testing (as

quality is determined by clinical situation according to postu-
late (1)).

(3) All analytical processes are monitored by a universal quality
     assurance network with traceability to SI units. (This
     requirement applies equally well to the central laboratory and
     the patient's home, with appropriately adjusted structures).

(4) Decentralization, as a process, requires steering by both the
     health agency and the profession.

(5) Decentralized clinical testing requires supervision by the
     profession.

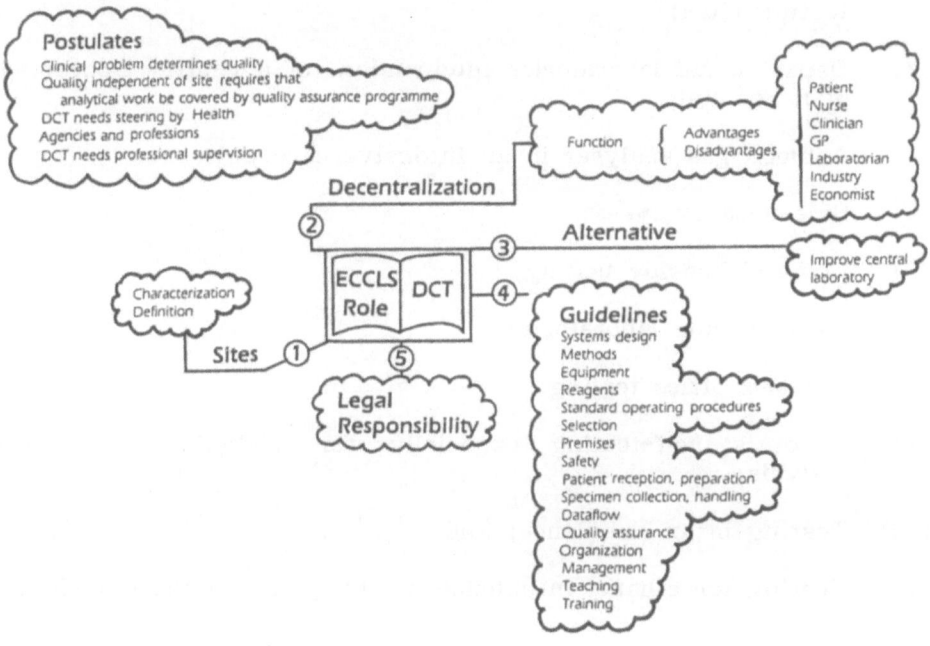

**Figure 18.2   Postulates and mind map of the possible role of
ECCLS in formulating requirements and guidelines for decentralized
clinical testing (DCT).**
Q.Ass. = quality assurance; DC = decentralization; HA = health
agencies; P = profession; GP = general practitioner.

THE PATIENT AND DECENTRALIZED TESTING

SITES

Before useful guidelines can be formulated, it is necessary to define what is meant by decentralized clinical testing sites and their respective characteristics. The list is long and diverse, ranging from sites with high professional competence available to those with none at all:

(1) The satellite laboratory of a hospital, managed as an integral part of the central laboratory, is hardly a decentralized unit in the functional sense;

(2) The 'central' laboratory of a small hospital with moderate specialization may lack academically educated professional expertise and therefore faces the problems of decentralized testing sites;

(3) Departmental laboratories independent of a central laboratory of a hospital;

(4) A blood gas analyser in an intensive care unit;

(5) Side-room analyses;

(6) Hospital bedside testing;

(7) Small private laboratories;

(8) Doctor's office testing;

(9) Patient's self-testing especially for diabetics and home dialysis;

(10) Testing in an ambulance; and

(11) Testing for ethanol in exhaled air by police at the roadside.

INFORMATION

For each type of decentralized testing site, each type of test, and each clinical situation an effort should be made to define and measure the functional, managerial and economic problems, and the pros and cons of decentralizing versus centralizing the analytical process. Opinions should be sought from patients, nursing staff, hospital clinicians, practitioners, laboratory staff, health agencies, industry and economists.

ADVANTAGES OF DECENTRALIZED TESTING

The advantages as seen from different viewpoints comprise a diversity of items:

(1)   Measuring the patient's properties in the clinically relevant situation as regards time and environmental and physiological conditions, including the medical emergency;

(2)   Producing results during the given physician-patient contact for rapid medical decision, including further testing with optimum testing sequence;

(3)   Saving patient's travel or transport, especially from remote areas;

(4)   Saving time of health personnel;

(5)   Saving transport of specimens, avoiding costs and deterioration;

(6)   Minimizing bureaucracy with forms, misunderstandings, delays, and mistaken identity;

(7)   Improving psychological factors by increasing the patient's insight into the disease process, self-responsibility for treatment, and familiarity with the testing situation. The patient suffers less anxiety due to waiting for an answer, and the practitioner gains satisfaction from a timely and self-managed decision-making process;

(8)   Increasing profit to institution or practitioner under some reimbursement schemes.

It is readily seen that the above advantages do not apply equally to all combinations of site, test, and clinical situation.

DISADVANTAGES OF DECENTRALIZED TESTING

The disadvantages or problems in some cases clearly overwhelm the advantages, whilst in others they may be accepted or counter-measures can be devised. The following may serve as a checklist of points to ponder:

(1)   Lower and sometimes clinically unacceptable quality in the form of higher analytical disturbance, both as regards its dispersion and location, leading to incomparability with other results and poorer diagnostic aid as well as more false negative dangerous results and expensive false positives.

The reasons may be inexperienced personnel, unsuited patient preparation and specimen collection, equipment or reagent insufficiency, lack of quality assurance, unsupervised selection of equipment, unsuitable equipment manuals, unsuitable method selection, poor procedure manuals and difficult up-dating, insufficient instrument maintenance and repair, unsuitable laboratory climate, reagent or specimen storage problems, difficult back-up, or less possibility of measuring the relevant quantity;

(2) Higher direct costs per result due to higher price of reagents, many smaller devices used by many operatives at many sites, small series, and more false positive results. Compensating possible indirect cost savings, for example in time and inconvenience, are often difficult to convert realistically into currency by suitable utility factors;

(3) Time consumption for analysis;

(4) Less supervision by professionals makes interpretation of both ambiguous or unexpected results and of clinical meaning more difficult;

(5) Equipment, reagents and manuals designed for laboratorians may not suit inexperienced personnel or patients;

(6) Difficulties of ensuring safety and health of patient, personnel, and surroundings may be due to inexperienced personnel, unsuitable premises or problems of decontamination and disposal;

(7) More problems of two-way information, data flow, and record keeping;

(8) Difficulties in achieving the needed major effort of education and continued training;

(9) Psychological problems of self-responsibility for patients functioning as analysts and therapists, and for inexperienced personnel operating with marginal knowledge;

(10) Legal responsibilities are not clear.

ALTERNATIVES TO DECENTRALIZED TESTING

In some cases a closer examination of a perceived need for decentralized testing shows that the claims for immediacy, urgency, and savings of cost and time are unreliable, or that the central laboratory can offer a clinically acceptable and cost-efficient solution by changing duty structure, equipment, method, specimen transport or data transfer. Such possibilities should always be explored to avoid the disadvantages listed above and may constitute an alternative or supplement to decentralization.

SUBJECTS IN NEED OF GUIDELINES

From the Conference papers and discussions it would appear that the health agencies, industry and professions should cooperate in preparing guidelines for a number of aspects of decentralized testing relevant to defined types of site. The following themes should be considered:

(1) Set of types of quantities that are suitable for decentralization,
(2) Clinical requirements of pre-analytical and analytical qualities, and predictive values,
(3) Requirements of analytical systems including methods, equipment, and reagents,
(4) Selection of procedure,
(5) Standard operating procedures,
(6) Premises and operational units,
(7) Safety requirements and health,
(8) Patient reception and preparation,
(9) Specimen collection and handling,
(10) Information and data flow,
(11) Quality assurance, comprising internal quality control, external quality assessment, consultative expert service, and supervision,
(12) Organization and management,
(13) Teaching and training, and
(14) Legal responsibilities.

Evidently, there is overlap between some of the listed areas, but that is not necessarily a disadvantage in moderate doses.

ECCLS'S ROLE IN PREPARING GUIDELINES

Given the present pressure to decentralize and the diverse and bewildering array of analytical devices being offered, the ECCLS has created a Standing Action Committee on Good Practice in Decentralized Clinical Laboratories (SAC). This body has set up seven subcommittees covering:

-   Reagents including reagent sets,
-   Quality requirements and quality assurance,
-   Premises and operational units,
-   Safety of personnel and environment,

THE PATIENT AND DECENTRALIZED TESTING

- Patient reception, preparation, and specimen handling,
- Data flow and contacts, and
- Management and organization.

In addition, an **Ad hoc Committee on Good Clinical Laboratory Management and Practice**, liaising with the SAC, is concerned with the broad guidelines of the Organization for Economic Cooperation and Development (OECD) that address central units of pharmaceutical testing rather than decentralized clinical testing, but might be modified by health authorities to apply to the clinical laboratory.

It will be seen that most if not all of the necessary guidelines may be created within the established framework.

Naturally, the documents should utilize existing recommendations from international and national sources, notably those emerging from the National Committee for Clinical Laboratory Standards' (NCCLS) Task Force on Decentralized Laboratories aiming at the physician's office laboratory.